1085 (4.50)

42,00

9³ 7.50 ~~7.50~~

medical
5110R

1.8

ANATOMY OF THE CENTRAL NERVOUS SYSTEM IN REVIEW

ANATOMY OF THE CENTRAL NERVOUS SYSTEM IN REVIEW

by

Donald H. Ford

Department of Anatomy, Downstate Medical Center, State University of New York, New York, U.S.A.

ELSEVIER SCIENTIFIC PUBLISHING COMPANY
AMSTERDAM — OXFORD — NEW YORK 1975

ELSEVIER SCIENTIFIC PUBLISHING COMPANY
335 Jan van Galenstraat
P.O. Box 211, Amsterdam, The Netherlands

AMERICAN ELSEVIER PUBLISHING COMPANY, INC.
52 Vanderbilt Avenue
New York, New York 10017

Library of Congress Card Number: 72-83204

ISBN 0-444-41025-2

Printed in The Netherlands

PREFACE

A knowledge of the structural organization of the central nervous system in conjunction with an understanding of its supporting meningeal envelopes and vascular supply is basic to the practice of neurology, neurosurgery and neuropathology. The question which often arises, however, is how much is needed for even these medical specialities. Too often the textbook writer is tempted to expand the information provided, particularly in those areas where he has a special interest. The resultant text is perhaps then unnecessarily complicated for any but the specialist in neuroscience. While most texts of neuroanatomy accept the need for adequate illustration, the more popular "reviews" of neuroanatomical structure tend toward an outline presentation. In view of the generally accepted difficulty experienced by students in conceptualizing brain organization, the omission of pictorial material seems unfortunate.

The aim of the author of the review is to provide both an outline and a pictorial (or schematic) survey of those aspects of the central nervous system which seem relevant to comprehending the basic function of the nervous system. This includes the major aspects of embryological development, gross structural divisions, internal and external support, vascular-ventricular systems, the structure of the functional unit (the neuron), the sensory and motor tract systems, as well as some indication of those changes occurring during maturation and aging. To some degree the information provided in this manner may be adequate for some of the shorter "core" courses. A short section of case histories is included to enable the student to attempt to utilize his anatomical information in relation to disorders of brain function. Thus, this review should enable a student to assess his fundamental knowledge of the gross and microscopic organization of the central nervous system and apply it to understanding those neurologic disorders which demonstrate symptoms related to dysfunction of specific structures.

Donald H. Ford

CONTENTS

Chapter 1

EMBRYOLOGY AND NEUROGENESIS

The tissue of origin of the central nervous system (CNS) is the neural ectoderm on the dorsal surface of the developing embryo. At the end of just three weeks of life, the embryo is a more-or-less oval disc about 1.5 cm long (Fig. 1). The long axis is related to the primitive streak in the posterior aspect of the embryonic disc and to the notochord rostrally. The notochord attaches rostrally to the prochordal plate of mesoderm, beneath the ectoderm.

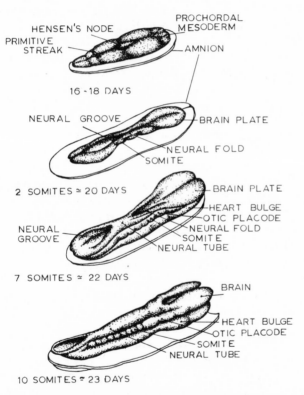

Fig. 1. The developing embryo, illustrating the position of Hensen's node from which the notochord develops by invagination. Note the formation of the neural tube which starts to fuse first in its middle portion. The rostral end gives rise to the brain plate, the remainder forming the spinal cord. The tube will remain open at both ends for some time, the openings being the anterior and posterior neuropores.

A. The CNS forms in relation to two structures.

1. Primitive streak — a posterior longitudinal thickened region.

2. Notochord — this tubular structure results from an ectodermal invagination starting at Hensen's node, which extends to the prochordal mesoderm.

B. The presence of the notochord and the prochordal mesoderm is believed to be necessary to induce the thickening of the overlying ectoderm to form the neural plate.

1. Increased cell division in the neural plate region leads to a thickening which finally infolds to form a neural groove (Figs 1 and 2), which can still be partially present at the two-somite stage at about 20 days. As the groove deepens, the edges merge and start to fuse along the midportion of the groove forming the neural tube. This process continues until the groove is closed except at the rostral and caudal ends. These openings are called the anterior and posterior neuropores. Further, as this growth occurs, there is a greater degree of development at the rostral end (cephalization) to form the cranial or brain portion of the CNS. The process by which this tube is formed is neurulation.

2. As the neural tube begins to close, it separates away from the adjacent ectoderm and sinks beneath it.

3. At the time of closure of the neural groove to form the neural tube, some cells along the margin of the tube separate away from the ectoderm to form two longitudinal columns of cells which run parallel to the neural tube. These are the neural crest columns (Fig. 2) which give rise to the dorsal root ganglia, autonomic ganglion cells, adrenomedullary cells, and the Schwann sheath cells, which form the myelin coverings of the peripheral nerves.

4. By about the 23rd day a definite brain structure has formed from the brain plate region of the neural tube.

5. The sequence of steps in the formation of the neural tube, neural crest, ganglia and peripheral nerves is illustrated in Fig. 2.
   a. Note that by stage D there are three well-developed zones (labelled in stage E).
      (i) Ependymal layer — the neuroepithelial germinative zone which gives rise to neurons and macroglia.
      (ii) Mantle layer — forms the grey matter of the spinal cord and primitive neural tube and is formed by migration of cells from the

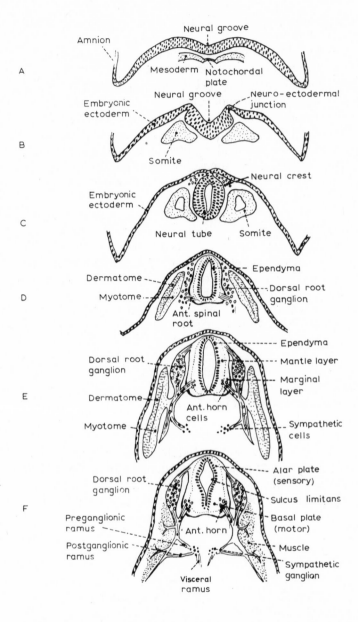

Fig. 2. A series of cross-sections through the developing neural tube illustrating the changes occurring, starting with the thickening of the ectoderm overlying the notochord to form a neural plate, neural groove and tube and its subsequent division into three layers. The neural crest cells which arise from the lateral margins of the neural ectoderm as the neural tube becomes pinched off are shown giving rise to dorsal root and autonomic ganglion units.

germinal layer. Further differentiation of neurons will proceed in the mantle layer.

(iii) Marginal layer — forms a peripheral region into which nerve fibers project in the spinal cord and primitive neural tube.

b. As the brain develops this primitive picture is altered in many areas of the brain so that the cross-sectional distribution of neurons in the mantle layer and nerve fibers in the marginal layer becomes greatly modified.

c. Differential rates of cell division lead to the formation of a pair of longitudinally oriented plates of cells, the alar and basal plates, which are separated by a thin furrow or sulcus, the sulcus limitans (Fig. 2F and Fig. 6). Dorsally, the two alar plates are joined by a roof plate and ventrally the two basal plates are joined by a floor plate.

C. The primary and secondary vesicles.

1. As a result of differential rates of cell proliferation at the rostral end of the neural tube, three distinct enlargements are formed (Fig. 3). These are the primary vesicles which are apparent by the 4th week.
   a. Prosencephalon (forebrain).
   b. Mesencephalon (midbrain).
   c. Rhombencephalon (hindbrain).

2. Secondary vesicles start to form by the end of the 4th week.
   a. Dorsolateral outgrowths occur from the rostral end of the prosencephalon. These are the telencephalic vesicles which will form the cerebral hemispheres. The remainder of the prosencephalon forms the diencephalon.
   b. The mesencephalon remains undivided.
   c. The rhombencephalon becomes subdivided into a rostral metencephalon, which gives rise to the cerebellum and pons. The caudal portion forms the myelencephalon or medulla oblongata.
   d. The remainder of the neural tube becomes the spinal cord (medulla spinalis).

3. Further development of the secondary vesicles leads to the formation of a brain which closely resembles that of the adult by the 13th to 14th week of development. It is, however, essentially devoid of the sulci which divide its surface into gyri. It is also apparent that the prosencephalic portion (telencephalon-diencephalon) is bent forward from the rest of the neural tube structures at an angle of 90° at its junction with the mesencephalon. This is the result of a series of complex movements or flexures which occur in the neural tube during its development.

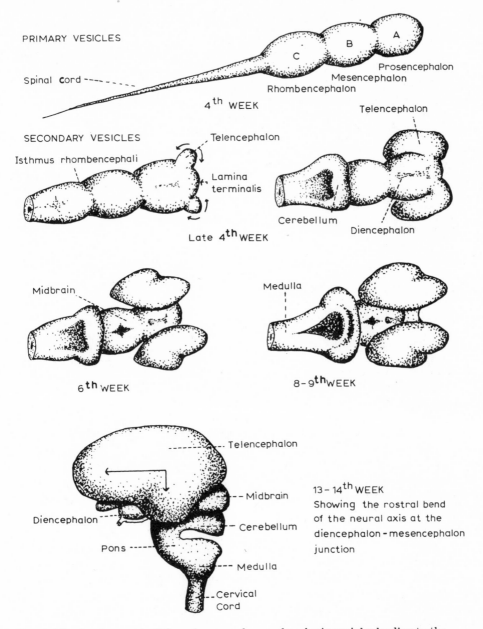

PRIMARY VESICLES

Spinal cord ---- - ---

B

C

A

Prosencephalon

Mesencephalon

Rhombencephalon

4th WEEK

SECONDARY VESICLES

Isthmus rhombencephali

Telencephalon

Lamina terminalis

Cerebellum

Telencephalon

Diencephalon

Late 4th WEEK

Midbrain

6th WEEK

Medulla

8-9th WEEK

Telencephalon

Midbrain

Diencephalon

Cerebellum

Pons

Medulla

Cervical Cord

13 - 14th WEEK
Showing the rostral bend
of the neural axis at the
diencephalon - mesencephalon
junction

Fig. 3. The development of the primary and secondary brain vesicles leading to the establishment of the telencephalon, diencephalon, mesencephalon, cerebellum, pons and medulla oblongata.

5

D. Flexures of the neural tube.

1. During growth, various kinks or flexures occur in the neural tube. These depend on the fact that (1) the neural tube is anchored at two points — the buccopharyngeal membrane (BPM in Fig. 4) and in the region of the cervical somites (S); and (2) that there is rapid growth of the rostral end of the neural tube which is not equivalent along its dorsal and ventral margins. A rather general depiction of these flexures is illustrated by Fig. 5.

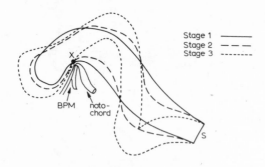

Stage 1 ————
Stage 2 — — —
Stage 3 --------

Fig. 4. A diagrammatic representation of the neural tube showing the changes in its relative position during the period in which the various flexures or bending of the neural tube occur. The bending of the tube appears to be due to two factors. One, the rapid growth that is occurring; two, that the tube is fixed at two points — the buccopharyngeal membrane (BPM) and in the region of the cervical somites (S).

a. Starting at the 3rd week, rapid growth rostrally and dorsally bends the tube rostrally to form a cephalic or mesencephalic flexure and caudally to form a cervical flexure.

b. During the 5th week there is a reverse bend into the pontine flexure.

c. Eventually all but the mesencephalic flexure disappear, leaving the brain bent forward at a 90° angle at the mesencephalic-diencephalic junction.

E. Regional development.

1. Spinal cord (medulla spinalis).

a. During the early phases of development the neural tube is essentially a hollow structure with a pseudostratified ependymal neuroepithelial germinative zone, a mantle region into which newly formed cells arising from the germinative layer will migrate and undergo differentiation, and a rather undifferentiated marginal layer (Fig. 2). Spongioblast cells derived from the germinal layer provide for processes which extend from the germinal cell surface to the outer surface of the neural tube. Expansions of the processes internally and externally form internal and external limiting membranes which provide an initial support for the neural tube.

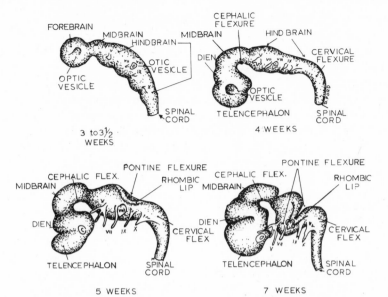

Fig. 5. A lateral view of the developing neural tube illustrating its appearance during the period in which the flexures occur.

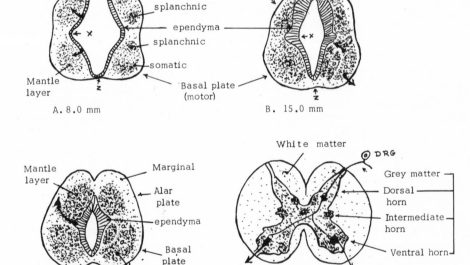

Fig. 6. A series of cross-sectional diagrams of the spinal cord illustrating the changes which occur from about five weeks of age at the 8.0 mm stage through to the terminal stage. x, sulcus limitans; y, roof plate; z, floor plate; DRG, dorsal root ganglion cell.

The appearance of the spinal cord in cross-section at the 8.0 mm stage (about five weeks) is characteristic of much of the neural tube with two pairs of longitudinally oriented plates of nerve and supporting elements (Fig. 6).

(i) Dorsolaterally — the alar plates (sensory in function) connected by a bridging roof plate.

(ii) Ventrolaterally — the basal plates (motor in function) connected by a bridging floor plate.

(iii) The sulcus limitans — (overlies a region of slower cell division) the longitudinal groove separating the alar and basal plates. It extends as far rostrally as the caudal margin of the diencephalon.

b. As cell division continues, increasing the neuronal and supporting cell populations, the alar and basal plates bulge internally, filling in the hollow portion of the neural tube dorsally and ventrally. The longitudinal masses of these primitive plates undergo a secondary longitudinal subdivision such that the most dorsal and ventral columns are associated with the somatic sensory-motor systems while the two intermediate cell columns become associated with the splanchnic sensory-motor system. The sulcus limitans, which separates the dorsal sensory from the ventral motor plates, persists for some time, but is gradually obliterated as the central canal shrinks, except in the region of the myelencephalon and metencephalon where it persists in the adult. The basal plate column becomes further subdivided into longitudinal arrays of cells (Fig. 6, 35 mm) which are associated with different muscle groups (i.e. flexors, extensors, abductors, adductors). Some of those in the region of the sulcus limitans fall into an intermediate group, which provides for various sorts of internuncial neurons.

Other neurons from the dorsal part of the ventral column of cells (a') will give rise to the intermediolateral cell column (sympathetic preganglionic neurons) of the adult. The cells located in the b column (Fig. 6C) produce axons which will be commissural and extend to the other side of the cord. At birth, the spinal cord resembles the adult cord in that the mantle layer forms an H-shaped column of cells surrounded by fibers in the marginal layer. The central canal is present at birth, but may be obliterated in the adult by overgrowth of glial cells surrounding the canal.

In these early developmental stages the emphasis appears to be directed toward the emergence of cells which will become neurons. Although numerous glial elements are formed, the major period of gliogenesis is postnatal, associated in part with myelinogenesis. Eventually, about 90% of the cell population of the CNS will consist of glial cells. While almost all neurons in man are formed early in embryonic development, numerous small granule cell elements will be formed postnatally, particularly in the hippocampus and cerebellum. Further, some cerebellar stellate and basket cells will be formed postnatally.

2. Myelencephalon (medulla oblongata).

a. The medulla starts initially with a structure resembling the spinal cord (Fig. 7, 10 mm) with the same separation of alar and basal plates into somatic and visceral (splanchnic), sensory and motor columns. However, as growth proceeds with extension of the basal plates towards each other and obliteration of the floor plate, the dorsal alar plates begin to extend out laterally, stretching out the roof plate (as in stages 2 and 3 in Fig. 7). Thus the roof plate becomes quite thin and consists of virtually nothing but the ependymal cell layer plus an investment of the supporting leptomeningeal tissues which surround the CNS. In this case it is the pia mater. By the 73 mm stage (between 12 and 16 weeks of age) this thin roof plate membrane becomes invaginated by blood vessels to form a choroid plexus.

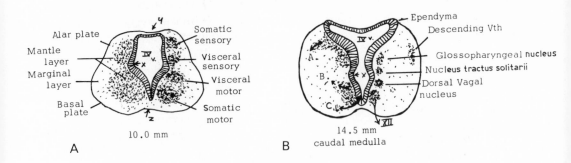

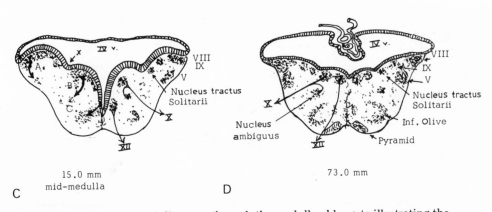

Fig. 7. A series of cross-sectional diagrams through the medulla oblongata illustrating the developmental changes occurring from an age of about 5½ weeks to a period between 12 and 16 weeks of age of gestation. A, cells from alar plate for trigeminal nuclei; B, cells from basal plate for nucleus ambiguus of the vagus; C, cells from ependyma migrating to form inferior olivary complex; x, sulcus limitans; y, roof plate; z, floor plate.

9

b. The lateral displacement of the alar plates enlarges this region of the hollow central canal into a large space or ventricular cavity. This is the fourth ventricle (IV v.) which, like the central canal and other of its more rostral dilations in the CNS, will be filled with a watery fluid, the cerebrospinal fluid.

c. The longitudinal columns of neurons of the alar and basal plates become the nuclei of origin or termination of various cranial nerves (descending trigeminal, V; vestibulocochlear, VIII; glossopharyngeal, IX; vagus, X; accessory, XI; and hypoglossal, XII).

d. Both alar and basal plates are believed to give rise to cells which will form the various reticular nuclei and the inferior olivary and arcuate nuclei (Fig. 7, stages 3 and 4).

3. Metencephalon (pons and cerebellum).

a. The pons consists of two parts. A dorsal tegmental portion which resembles the medulla and a basal portion which contains descending fiber systems and cells whose axons project to the cerebellum. The dorsal pontine

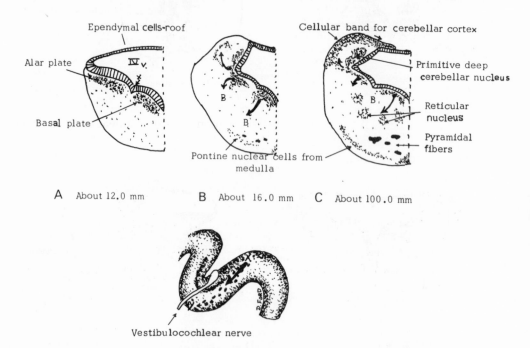

A   About 12.0 mm   B   About 16.0 mm   C   About 100.0 mm

Vestibulocochlear nerve

Fig. 8. A series of cross-sectional figures illustrating the developmental changes occurring in the pons from about 6 weeks of age to about 16 weeks of age. The lower figure illustrates the migration of cells from the dorsolateral aspect of the medulla oblongata (X) to the region of the basal pons (Y), providing for neurons of the basal pons. A, cells migrating from alar plate to form cerebellar cortex; B, cells migrating from alar and basal plates to form pontine reticular nuclei, including also cells from the basal plate.

10

portion of the metencephalon (Fig. 8) resembles the medulla at the 10—12 mm stage, showing the same lateral outgrowth of the alar plates and fusion of the basal plates ventrally. As in the medulla the sulcus limitans persists, separating alar and basal plates. Motor cell groups giving rise to the abducens (VI) and facial (VII) cranial nerve nuclei are found in this region in the adult. However, they develop originally in the medulla and are shifted rostrally during the formation of the pontine flexure and remain in a rostral pontine location when the pontine flexure straightens out. The same is true for the rostral portion of the VIIIth nerve vestibular nuclear group which also originates in the medulla. The only cranial nerve components which are actually derived in the pons are the motor and main sensory nuclei of the trigeminal nerve and a part of the trigeminal descending nucleus. At least some of the cells of the basal pons migrate from the dorsolateral aspect of the medulla oblongata during development (Fig. 8) to assume a position at the base of the metencephalon. It is not clear if all the cells of these nuclear groups are derived in this fashion. These cells will eventually receive terminals from cells in the cerebral cortex and they will direct their own axons to the cerebellar cortex.

    (i) Reticular formation nuclei in the metencephalon are probably derived from both alar and basal plates.

    b. The cerebellum is derived from alar plate cells which collect to form a laterally placed structure, the rhombic lip (Fig. 9). One group of cells is believed to migrate dorsomedially from the region of the lateral recess of the fourth ventricle close to the roof plate to form the deep nuclei of the cerebellum (Fig. 8, 100 mm). Other cells also located in the lateral recesses give rise to the large Purkinje cells. Another body of cells which does not appear to differentiate also arises from the lateral recess and moves through the rudimentary cerebellum to form an external granule cell layer. Some cells also appear to migrate into what will be the internal granule cell layer.

    (i) The external granule cell layer deserves additional comment because it is one of the areas of the CNS where cell division has been observed to occur for appreciable periods after birth. The first cells which migrate from this layer following cell division of the germinal elements are the basket cells. Next are the stellate cells of the molecular layer. Finally, the remaining granule cells in the external layer migrate past the Purkinje cells to the internal granule cell layer.

    (ii) Note that the rhombic lip extends out laterally to the lateral apex of the fourth ventricle at which point the cells of the rhombic lip giving rise to the cerebellum are in juxtaposition with caudally placed cells which give rise to the vestibular nuclear centers. This common point of origin may help explain the close association of the vestibular and cerebellar systems.

    c. After the cellular bands which overgrow the roof plate meet in what will be the cerebellar vermis, the cerebellar hemispheres begin to grow out laterally (Fig. 9, 56—60 mm, about 12 weeks of age). Note that the develop-

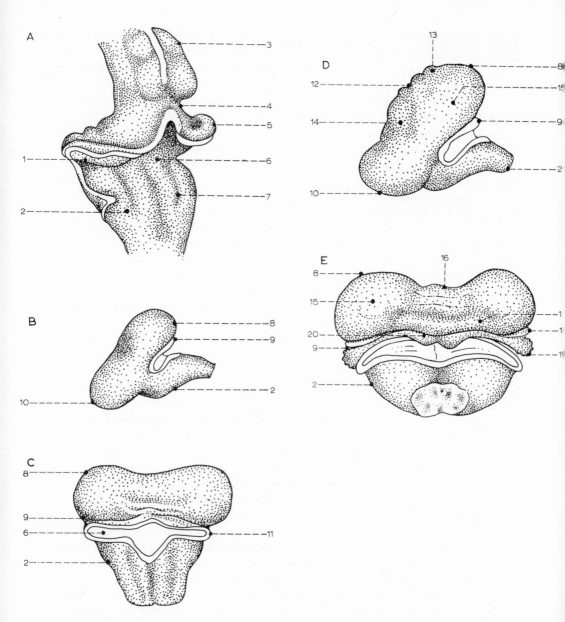

Fig. 9. A series of figures illustrating the changes occurring in the cerebellum. The state of development shown in A is at about 7 weeks (17 mm). B and C represent a 56 mm embryo at about 12 weeks of age. The age at 112 mm is about 16 weeks of gestation (D, E). 1, primitive cerebellum; 2, medulla; 3, tectum mesencephali; 4, isthmus rhombencephali; 5, rhombic lip; 6, IVth ventricle; 7, sulcus limitans; 8, corpus cerebelli; 9, posterolateral fissure; 10, pons; 11, lateral recess; 12, primary fissure; 13, postclival fissure; 14, anterior lobe; 15, posterior lobe; 16, vermis; 17, tonsil; 18, paraflocculus; 19, flocculus; 20, nodulus. 20, nodulus.

12

ment of folia occurs first in the medial vermian region and then extends laterally.

(i) Peduncles. During the course of development, three pairs of peduncles become associated with the cerebellum.

(a) Inferior cerebellar peduncle (restiform body) which can be just recognized after about eight weeks as thin fibers arising from the spinal cord which extend rostrally into the alar plate to reach the cerebellum. Olivo- and reticulocerebellar fibers will also contribute to this bundle.

(b) Middle cerebellar peduncle (brachium pontis). These fibers arise from cells forming the basal pons.

(c) Superior cerebellar peduncle (brachium conjunctivum). This arises at about eight weeks of age as small scattered fibers, extending rostrally from the deep cerebellar nuclei into the mesencephalon.

4. Region of the isthmus rhombencephali.

a. The constriction between the primitive rhombencephalic (hindbrain) and mesencephalic (midbrain) vesicles where growth is less rapid than in the caudally and rostrally adjacent areas.

(i) Site of origin of the trochlear (IV) cranial nerve nucleus. Nerve fibers arising from the nucleus course dorsally to exit at the region of the isthmus, where the fibers decussate.

(ii) With further growth during the period of flexure formation (12 mm, 6 weeks of age), the cells forming the trochlear nucleus in the basal plate are pushed rostrally and come to lie in the mesencephalon in the adult. The nerve fibers, however, still exit at the isthmus.

(iii) Alar plate derivatives are also displaced rostrally during this same 12—16 mm period. Thus, a component of the trigeminal cranial nerve (V) comes to be in the alar plate region of the mesencephalon. This is the mesencephalic root of the trigeminal nerve.

5. Mesencephalon (midbrain) — starts with the same general appearance as the primitive spinal cord (Fig. 10, 23 mm). As growth of alar and basal plates continues, the central canal becomes somewhat less constricted than in the spinal cord. The remaining canal is known as the cerebral aqueduct.

a. Alar plate derivatives form the corpora quadrigemina or tectal plate.

(i) Superior colliculus, rostrally: characterized by a laminar cellular-fiber architecture (Fig. 10, 112 mm stage at left side of figure).

(ii) Inferior colliculus, caudally: characterized by a large rather homogeneous nucleus (Fig. 10, 112 mm stage, right side of figure).

b. The basal plate gives rise to the oculomotor nucleus (third cranial nerve), which is really a conglomerate of five separate nuclear groups, each for separate extraocular muscles.

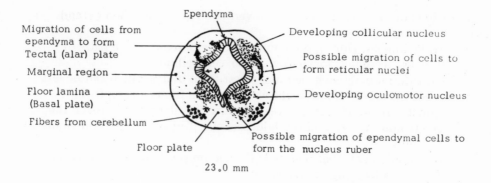

Ependyma

Migration of cells from ependyma to form Tectal (alar) plate

Developing collicular nucleus

Possible migration of cells to form reticular nuclei

Marginal region

Floor lamina (Basal plate)

Developing oculomotor nucleus

Fibers from cerebellum

Floor plate

Possible migration of ependymal cells to form the nucleus ruber

23.0 mm

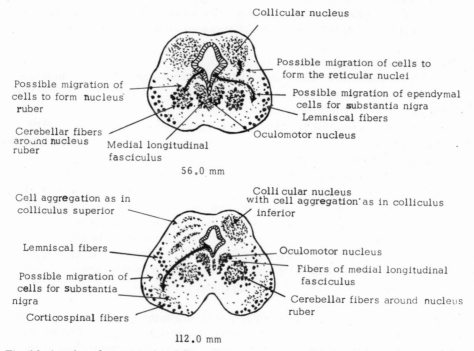

Collicular nucleus

Possible migration of cells to form nucleus ruber

Possible migration of cells to form the reticular nuclei

Possible migration of ependymal cells for substantia nigra

Lemniscal fibers

Cerebellar fibers around nucleus ruber

Medial longitudinal fasciculus

Oculomotor nucleus

56.0 mm

Cell aggregation as in colliculus superior

Collicular nucleus with cell aggregation as in colliculus inferior

Lemniscal fibers

Oculomotor nucleus

Fibers of medial longitudinal fasciculus

Possible migration of cells for substantia nigra

Cerebellar fibers around nucleus ruber

Corticospinal fibers

112.0 mm

Fig. 10. A series of cross-sectional figures illustrating the developmental changes occurring in the mesencephalon. x, sulcus limitans.

c. Reticular formation nuclei and the cells forming the central grey around the cerebral aqueduct are probably derived from both alar and basal plates. The precise origin of the cells forming the red nucleus (nucleus ruber) and substantia nigra is not clear.

d. Fiber tracts.

(i) Cerebellomesencephalothalamic fibers. These are first seen at about the 23 mm stage as fibers penetrating into the basal area.

14

(ii) Lemniscal fibers carrying sensory input to the thalamus and reticular formation are present by the 56 mm stage. These fibers are spread through the ventrolateral aspect of the alar plate and dorsolateral part of the basal plate during the third month. Cells of the substantia nigra come to be ventral in relation to the lemniscal fibers. Their precise origin is uncertain.

(iii) Cortical efferent fiber projections are apparent by the 112 mm stage (16 weeks). These are applied ventral to all the other components.

6. Prosencephalon (forebrain). This becomes divided into the telencephalon (cerebral hemisphere) and the diencephalon (Fig. 11).

a. The telencephalon develops as an outpocketing from the rostral end of the prosencephalon and extends from the dorsolateral aspect, taking a portion of the roof plate with it as it grows out.

b. The optic evagination occurs ventrolaterally from the portion which will form the diencephalon. The curved inferior portion of the diencephalon possesses a rounded prominence which continues laterally with the posterior inferior wall of the optic cup. This will be the site of the optic chiasm at birth. The hollow central canal forms a fourth ventricle caudally, and the cerebral aqueduct in the midbrain becomes compressed mediolaterally in the region of the diencephalon to form the third ventricle. Lateral extensions continue into the cerebral hemisphere, forming the lateral ventricles. There is also an extension of this fluid-filled cavity into the optic sac evaginations.

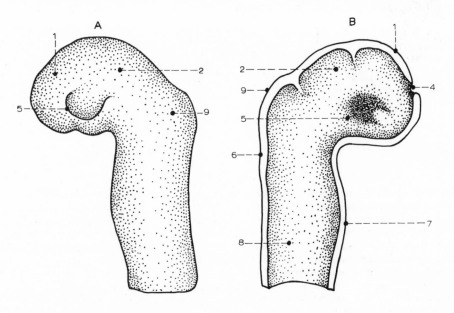

(Fig. 11, continued overleaf.)

15

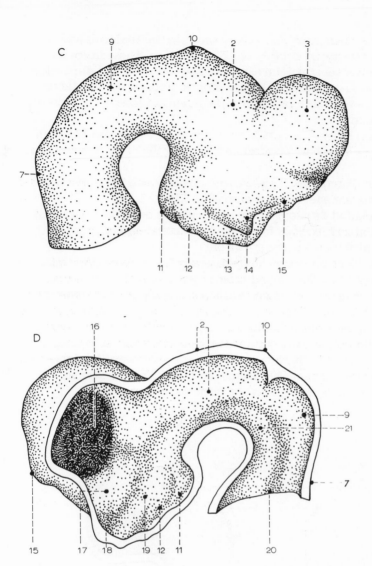

Fig. 11. A series of diagrams illustrating the appearance of the forebrain structures from the medial and lateral aspects at 3½ weeks (A, B; 2.5 mm stage) and at about 5½ weeks (C, D; 10.2 mm stage) of age. Note that there is a remnant of the anterior neuropore still present at 3½ weeks. Observe by 5½ weeks of age that there are indications foreshadowing the hypophysis, visual system and that a cerebral hemisphere is clearly discernible.
1, pallial region; 2, diencephalon; 3, telencephalon; 4, anterior neuropore; 5, optic evagination; 6, isthmus rhombencephali; 7, pons; 8, medulla; 9, midbrain; 10, pineal region; 11, mammillary region; 12, tuber cinereum; 13, hypophyseal pouch; 14, optic stalk; 15, olfactory lobe; 16, foramen of Monro; 17, corpus striatum; 18, optic recess; 19, hypothalamus; 20, sulcus limitans; 21, basal plate.

16

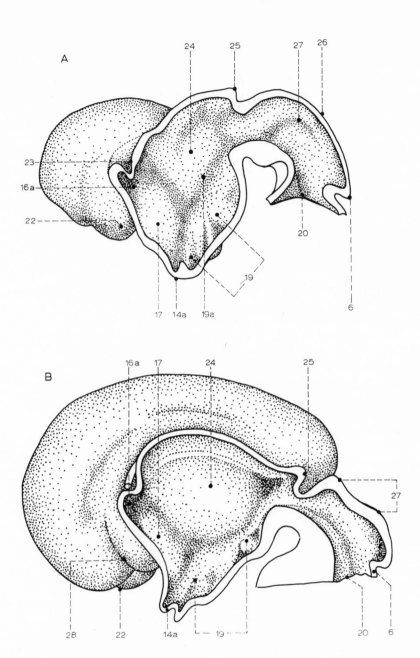

Fig. 12. The continued development of the prosencephalon through ages of about 6 weeks (A, 13.6 mm stage) until slightly older than 12 weeks (B, 60.0 mm stage), as seen from the medial aspect, to illustrate the changes occurring in the diencephalon. 6, isthmus rhombencephali; 14a, optic chiasm; 16a, interventricular foramen; 19, hypothalamus; 20, sulcus limitans; 22, rhinencephalon; 23, choroid fissure; 24, thalamus; 25, pineal; 26, mesencephalon; 27, corpora quadrigemina; 28, hippocampal fissure.

c. As seen from the medial aspect, the diencephalon develops into two major regions, the dorsal thalamus and the ventrally placed hypothalamus (Fig. 12, 13.6 mm between 6 and 7 weeks, and 60 mm at about 12 weeks of age). Due to regional differences in the rate of cell proliferation, a sulcus (hypothalamic sulcus) appears between these two regions. In the dorsal thalamus there are additional subdivisions, one of which can be seen in the midsagittal plane.

(i) Epithalamus. This midline structure starts as two proliferative zones on the dorsal aspect of the diencephalon, just rostral to the midbrain. These two zones fuse to form a parenchymal structure, the pineal or epiphysis. Just rostral to the pineal another small nuclear group forms on each side, the habenular nucleus. Two longitudinal striae, the striae medullares thalami, are also incorporated in this subdivision.

(ii) Other diencephalic centers develop which cannot be seen on the midsagittal plane. These form

(a) The metathalamus, which is comprised of the medial and lateral geniculate bodies.

(b) The subthalamus, which is comprised of the subthalamic nucleus and a region which will later be referred to as the zona incerta, with its related fiber bundles. This is not generally considered as part of the dorsal thalamus or hypothalamus.

d. The space between the two diencephalic masses is the third ventricle. It can be seen to be connected laterally through the interventricular foramen (foramen of Monro) with the lateral ventricles, which are the fluid-filled spaces of the cerebral hemispheres. Just rostral and ventral to the foramen another nuclear mass bulges into the third ventricle. This is the corpus striatum, which gives rise to the putamen, globus pallidus, caudate nucleus and amygdala of the adult.

e. The cerebral hemisphere is observed to expand rostrally, dorsally and caudally in a rapid manner. By the 13.6 mm stage a well-defined structure begins to bulge out medially at the rostral inferior aspect, just anterior to the corpus striatum. This is the rhinencephalon (smell brain), which becomes the hippocampus of the adult brain. The hippocampal fissure, which separates this rather primitive part of the cortex from phylogenetically newer areas is clearly apparent by the 60 mm stage.

As seen from the lateral aspect, the cerebral hemisphere evolves quite rapidly into a form comparable to that seen in the adult (Fig. 13). The lateral fissure (Sylvian fissure) is in evidence by the 16th week, while by 32 weeks slight indentations denoting the other sulci are apparent. The lateral fissure and the central sulcus (of Rolando) are the two demarcations which seem to be primary in establishing what would be the adult pattern of sulci laterally. Medially, the first sulcal grooves to appear are the hippocampal, cingulate, parieto-occipital and calcarine. By birth, all the major sulci of the adult brain are readily apparent and the expanded lateral fissure has closed over to

18

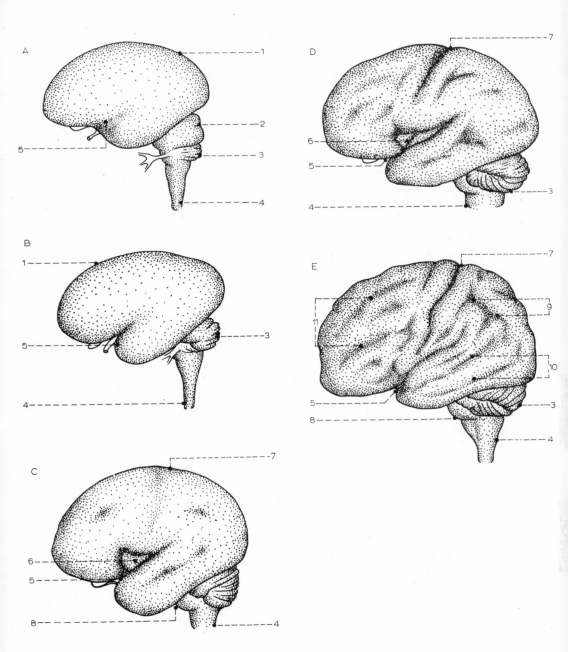

Fig. 13. A series of diagrams illustrating the lateral aspect of the cerebral hemispheres to demonstrate the development of gyri from about 11 weeks postconception until birth. (Adapted from Patten's *Human Embryology*, 1953.) A, 11 weeks; B, 16—17 weeks; C, 24—26 weeks; D, 32—34 weeks; E, newborn. 1, telencephalon; 2, mesencephalon; 3, cerebellum; 4, medulla; 5, developing lateral fissure; 6, insula; 7, sulcus centralis; 8, pons; 9, parietal sulci; 10, temporal sulci; 11, frontal sulci.

19

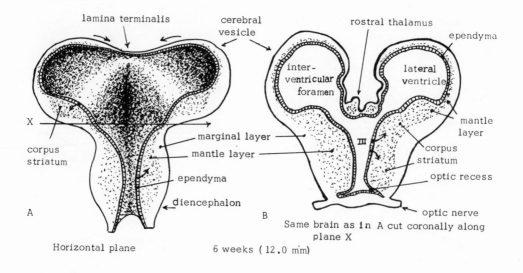

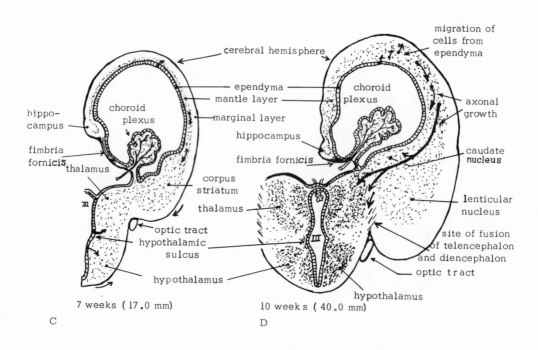

Fig. 14. A series of diagrams of sections of the prosencephalon demonstrating the outgrowth of the hemispheres from the rostral aspect of the prosencephalon (A). B, C and D illustrate sections in the coronal plane demonstrating the further outgrowth of the hemisphere upwards and then downwards lateral to the diencephalon (C and D).

conceal the underlying insula. When viewed in section (Fig. 14) the cerebral hemisphere appears first as a rather large saccular structure lined by ependyma. The proliferation of cells in this hemispheric sac is sufficiently extensive to fill in completely the space between the ependyma and the external limiting membrane, leaving no marginal layer. The first cell layer which is established is the deepest layer. Other cells arising from the ependyma then migrate through the deepest layer to form the next deepest and so on until the typical six-layered cortex of the adult is established. The axons from these cells are then directed medially. This serves to establish the position of the fibers which will become myelinated later as being deep to the grey matter instead of being superficial as they are in the spinal cord.

As the hemisphere enlarges, it grows downward towards the diencephalon (Fig. 14C and D) and fuses against it. The line of fusion appears to form a plane through which the corticofugal fibers will pass by about ten weeks of age, forming the internal capsule. Also, as these axons are directed away from the cortex toward lower centers, they pass in bundles through the corpus striatum, breaking it up into the nuclear groups seen in the adult. Other fibers

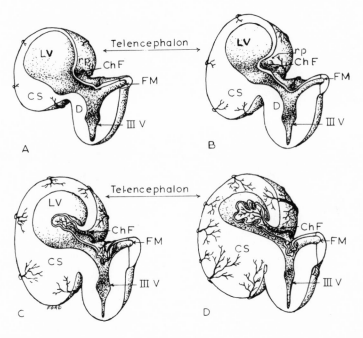

≈ 32- 44 DAYS (12 - 24 mm)

Fig. 15. A series of sections in the coronal plane illustrating the changes occurring in relation to the choroidal fissure (ChF) leading subsequently to the formation of a choroid plexus. CS, corpus striatum; D, diencephalon; FM, foramen of Monro; LV, lateral ventricle; rp, roof plate; III V, third ventricle.

21

arising from cells in the thalamus will utilize the same plane to proceed toward the cortex.

f. Fig. 15 depicts the growth of the hemisphere in a manner which illustrates that the roof plate of the prosencephalon extends out onto the medial aspect of the hemisphere as it becomes evaginated (A and B). As the hemisphere grows, upward and medially, this part of the roof plate (rp) becomes folded, forming the choroidal fissure (ChF). As development proceeds, vessels investing the layer of pia adjacent to the roof plate proliferate to form the choroid plexus of the lateral ventricle and, more medially, of the third ventricle as well.

g. When viewed from the lateral aspect, the corpus striatum may be seen to be forming in the floor of the telencephalic sac (Fig. 16). The large hollow cavity of the ventricle is dorsal to it. As development proceeds, the caudal part of the hemisphere grows downward and the forward, imparting a rather C-shaped appearance to the ventricle. At the same time the corpus striatum is expanding dorsally, accentuating this process. Finally, the corpus striatum is interdicted by fibers arising from the cortex which grow through it in such

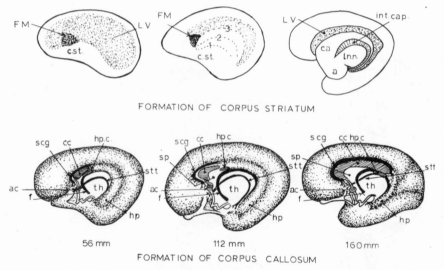

FORMATION OF CORPUS STRIATUM

FORMATION OF CORPUS CALLOSUM

56 mm   112 mm   160 mm

Fig. 16. The three diagrams at the top of the figure illustrate the upward growth of the corpus striatum (c.st.) during development which occurs at the same time as the hemisphere is extending upward, caudally and then inferiorly. Since the hemisphere is hollow, this series of extensions of the hemisphere, accompanied by the upgrowth of the corpus striatum, imparts a C shape to the lateral ventricle (LV) in the hemisphere. The numbers 1, 2 and 3 indicate successive levels of the corpus striatum. a, amygdala; FM, foramen of Monro; Ln.n, lenticular nucleus (putamen + globus pallidus). The lower three diagrams illustrate the formation of commissures. ac, anterior commissure; cc, corpus callosum; f, fornix; hp, hippocampus; hpc, hippocampal commissure; scg, supracallosal gyrus (hippocampal rudiment); sp, septum pellucidum; stt, stria terminalis; th, thalamus.

22

a way as to divide it into a number of subnuclear masses: caudate nucleus, lenticular nucleus (putamen and globus pallidus), and amygdala.

h. There are a number of commissural bundles which interconnect homologous regions of the cortex. They all start from a commissural plate which is in the region of the anterior commissure (ac) of the adult brain. At this time, the hippocampus extends up over the top of the third ventricle and is connected by a short bundle of fibers, the fornix (f) with the diencephalon (th). During development, some of the fibers arising from the cortex pass through this plate and are soon delineated into three major bundles, depending on the origin: those connecting the olfactory bulbs and amygdalar regions pass through the anterior commissure; those arising from the hippocampus pass through the hippocampal commissure; those connecting the great mass of the cerebral hemisphere pass through the corpus callosum (cc). The corpus becomes the largest of the commissures. As it enlarges, it pushes the hippocampal commissure caudally, shortening the mass of the hippocampus and lengthening the fiber bundle (fornix) which arises from it. One small part of the hippocampus is left adherent to the dorsum of the corpus callosum as the hippocampal rudiment of the supracallosal gyrus (scg). Fibers from the hippocampus extend through this gyrus to terminate just rostral to the corpus callosum.

F. Table of brain development in relation to age and crown—rump length*

Age in weeks	Crown—rump length (mm)	Brain development
2.5	1.5	Neural groove indicated.
3.5	2.5	Neural groove prominent, closing rapidly, neural crest a continuous band.
4.0	5.0	Neural tube closed, three primary vesicles of brain represented, nerves and ganglia forming, ependymal, mantle and marginal layers present.
5.0	8.0	Five brain vesicles, cerebral hemispheres bulging, nerves and ganglia better represented (suprarenal cortex accumulating).
6.0	12.0	Three primary flexures of brain represented, diencephalon large, nerve plexuses present, epiphysis recognizable, sympathetic ganglia forming segmental masses, meninges indicated.
7.0	17.0	Cerebral hemispheres becoming large, corpus striatum and thalamus prominent, infundibulum and Rathke's pouch in contact, choroid plexuses appearing, suprarenal medulla begins invading cortex.

Age in weeks	Crown—rump length (mm)	Brain development
8.0	23.0	Cerebral cortex begins to acquire typical cells, olfactory lobes visible, dura and pia-arachnoid distinct, chromaffin bodies appearing.
10.0	40.0	Spinal cord attains definitive internal structure.
12.0	56.0	Brain attains its general structural features, cord shows cervical and lumbar enlargement, cauda equina and filum terminale appearing, neuroglial types beginning to differentiate.
16.0	112.0	Hemispheres conceal much of brain stem, cerebral lobes delimited, corpora quadragemina appear, cerebellum assumes some prominence.
20—40	160—350	Commissures completed (20 weeks), myelinization in cord begins (20 weeks), cerebral cortex typically layered (25 weeks), cerebral fissures and convolutions appearing rapidly (28—30 weeks), myelinization of brain begins (36—40 weeks).

*From: L.B. Arey, *Developmental Anatomy*, 6th ed., W.B. Saunders Co., Philadelphia, p. 106, 1954.

G. Average weight of normal brains (infants and children)*

Age	Body length (cm)	Body weight (kg)	Brain weight (g)
Birth—3 days	49	3.4	335
3—7 days	49		358
1—3 weeks	52		382
3—5 weeks	52		413
5—7 weeks	53		422
7—9 weeks	55		489
3 months	56	6.5	516
4 months	59		540
5 months	61		644
6 months	62	8.5	660
7 months	65		691
8 months	65		714
9 months	67	9.8	750
10 months	69		809
11 months	70		852

Age	Body length (cm)	Body weight (kg)	Brain weight (g)
12 months	73	10.8	925
14 months	74		944
16 months	77		1010
18 months	78	12.2	1042
20 months	79		1050
22 months	82		1059
24 months	84	13.2	1064
3 years	88	15.2	1141
4 years	99	17.3	1191
5 years	106	19.4	1237
6 years	109	21.9	1243
7 years	113	24.6	1263
8 years	119	27.7	1273
9 years	125	31.0	1275
10 years	130	34.8	1290
11 years	135	38.8	1320
12 years	139	43.2	1351

*Modified from J.M. Coppoletta and S.B. Wolbach, Body lengths and normal weights of more important vital organs between birth and twelve years of age, *Am. J. Pathol.*, 9 (1933) 55—70, in O. Saphir, *Autopsy Diagnosis and Technic*, 4th ed., Paul B. Hoeber Inc., New York, 1946, p. 508.

H. Neurogenesis.

The process of neurogenesis which results in the formation of the cellular elements of the nervous system is reviewed in Fig. 17. During neurulation, the neural tube forms by invagination of the surface ectoderm to form the neural tube (A). In cross-section this appears as a simple epithelial tube of pseudostratified columnar cells. The entire central nervous system will develop from this tube. Elements of this germinal layer which remain do not migrate out into the mantle layer and will be retained as the ependymal layer in the adult. At the time of formation of the neural tube, cells adjacent to those which become invaginated form two longitudinal columns of cells parallel to the neural tube. These cells, which separate away from the surface ectoderm, are the neural crest cells.

A schematized illustration of the simple undifferentiated neural tube in cross-section is represented at A. At this time the tube is open at both ends and unrecognizable as a nervous system. A central hollow cavity is present which will be maintained through subsequent stages and finally becomes the ventricular system in the adult.

As a result of proliferation of cells in the germinal layer, the tube becomes thickened until finally three distinct layers may be discerned: ependymal, mantle and marginal. The mantle layer, in the region of the cord, represents the area into which neural and glial cells will migrate after formation in the

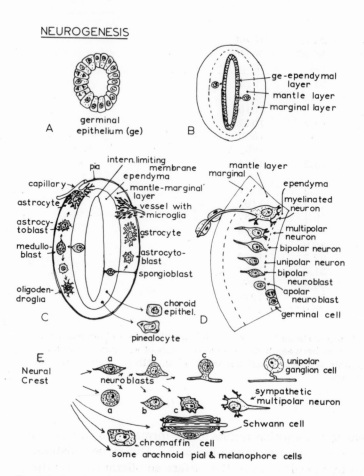

Fig. 17. A series of diagrams illustrating the derivation of the glial and neural elements from the germinal epithelium (ge). C represents the development of the supporting glial elements plus the choroidal epithelium and parenchymal pineal cells. D illustrates the formation of a multipolar neuron, while E illustrates the various cellular elements derived from the neural crest cells.

neuroepithelial germinal layer. The outermost marginal layer then becomes a region into which nerve fibers interconnecting various levels of the nervous system will project.

Part C of Fig. 17 illustrates the various supporting cell types which may be derived from the germinal epithelium. The left side of the figure illustrates some cells which form medulloblasts and give rise to either astrocytes or oligodendroglia in the adult form. Note that the astrocyte derived from the medulloblast is illustrated as having a relationship with an outer pial meningeal layer, with an inner ependymal layer, or with a capillary. Not illustrated is a fourth relationship; namely, with a neuron. The neuronal relationship may be with either the afferent or efferent processes of the neuron, as well as with the cell body, and may also occur in the white matter in relation solely to axons. This is true for any astrocytes, whether derived from medulloblasts or spongioblasts. The medulloblasts also give rise to the oligodendroglial cells.

Another cell type derived from the germinal layer which is concerned with internal support of the CNS is the spongioblast. This cell provides for internally and externally directed processes which become involved in the formation of the internal and external limiting membranes of the neural tube. The latter is just subjacent to the pia. Some of the elements will also become modified to form astrocytes. In the cerebrum the spongioblastic processes provide guidance fibers for externally migrating neuronal elements.

Four other supporting cell types evolve from the germinal epithelium in specialized areas of the CNS. The ependymal cells associated with the roof plate in the regions of the lateral, third and fourth ventricles become modified to form the epithelial cells of the choroid plexus (C in Fig. 17). The ependymal cells also are involved in the formation of the parenchymal and supporting cells of the pineal gland in the region of the caudal dorsal aspect of the third ventricle. The supporting cells are in all likelihood modified glial cells. The third category represents cells which are really modified ependymal cells. These are the cells of the subcommissural organ just beneath the posterior aspect of the third ventricle. They are believed to have a secretory activity in lower forms. A final category of supporting cells may yet be listed which may have some similarity to the cells of the subcommissural organ. These are the tanycytes which are also modified ependymal cells found at the inferior aspect of the third ventricle in relation to the tuber cinereum and may also have a secretory function. Ependymal cells in the adult are often ciliated and also may possess microvilli. They range from cuboidal to columnar in shape. Over white matter they are very low cuboidal elements.

Part D of Fig. 17 illustrates the various changes involved in the formation of a multipolar neuron from the germinal cells of the ependymal layer, progressing from a neuroblast to a fully formed myelinated adult neuron.

Cells of the neural crest (part E, Fig. 17) give rise to a wide variety of cell types. The sensory cells of the dorsal root ganglia and the motor neurons of the sympathetic ganglia are derived from these cells. They progress through a series of blast cells (a, b and c) which culminate in either mature unipolar ganglion cells or multipolar sympathetic neurons. The external supporting Schwann sheath cells of the peripheral nerves as well as the satellite cells of the sympathetic and dorsal root ganglia are derived from this component. Furthermore, there is evidence to indicate that at least some of the cells of the outer pial and arachnoid supporting layers of the CNS are formed from neural crest cells. Finally there are the chromaffin cells of the adrenal gland and the melanocytes found scattered throughout the leptomeninges.

Thus, the notochord and prochordal mesoderm induce changes in the dorsally adjacent ectoderm which lead to the formation of a neural tube and its associated neural crest element. From this primary tube and the crest cells all but one cell found in the nervous system will develop. This last cell type is the microglial cell, of uncertain true origin, but it is believed to be associated with the migration of vascular elements into the CNS. These cells may, as some believe, be derived from the pericytes which are located in the basement membranes of the capillaries of the CNS.

Chapter 2

A GENERAL SURVEY OF THE FUNCTIONAL CNS COMPONENTS

A. Medulla spinalis (spinal cord).

1. In the adult, the spinal cord extends from about the junction of the 1st and 2nd lumbar vertebrae to the foramen magnum where it is continuous with the medulla oblongata (Fig. 18).

a. Numerous fibers extend from the caudal end (conus medullaris) inferiorly to exit from the spinal canal at their appropriate intervertebral foramina. This large group of fibers forms the cauda equina. As one proceeds

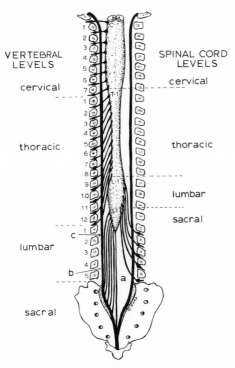

Fig. 18. A diagrammatic representation of the spinal cord within the spinal canal illustrating the relative difference between spinal cord segmental levels and vertebral levels. Note the dura attaches to the inner surface of the occipital bone at the level of the foramen magnum at the top of the figure, being separate from the periosteum throughout the spinal canal levels. a, subarachnoid space; b, epidural space; c, spinal dura mater. The levels of the cord are indicated as C-1 (cervical), T-1 (thoracic), L-1 (lumbar), and S-1 (sacral).

29

rostrally, the nerve fibers leave the cord at progressively less acute angles. Note that the segmental spinal cord levels do not match those of the vertebral bodies and that this discrepancy is most marked at sacral cord levels.

2. Comprised internally of an H-shaped core of grey matter containing the neuronal cell bodies (Fig. 19).

a. Dorsal horn (cornu posterius), associated with sensory relay functions. Fig. 19 shows some of the major subnuclear groups.

b. Ventral horn (cornu anterius), contains motor cells to innervate the trunk and appendicular musculature. These motor cells are organized in longitudinal columns such that there are distributions of cells for flexor, extensor, abductors, etc., muscles (Fig. 20).

c. There is a lateral horn (cornu laterale) of motor neurons extending from T_1 to L_2 or L_3 which provides for the preganglionic neurons of the sympathetic motor system for the innervation of visceral structures. Parasympathetic innervation of pelvic viscera is provided for by fibers arising from cord levels at S_2, S_3 and S_4.

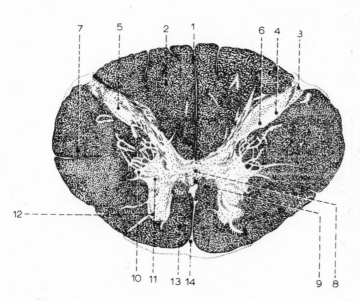

Fig. 19. A cross-section of the upper thoracic cord illustrating the dorsal, ventral and lateral horns (cornua posterius, laterale and anterius) as well as the intermediate grey (substantia grisea centralis and lateralis). The posterior, lateral and anterior funiculi are also illustrated. 1, posterior medial septum; 2, funiculus posterior; 3, tract of Lissauer; 4, substantia gelatinosa; 5, cornu posterius (sensory); 6, nucleus proprius of 5; 7, funiculus lateralis; 8, substantia grisea centralis; 9, commissura alba; 10, cornu laterale; 11, substantia grisea lateralis; 12, cornu anterius (motor); 13, funiculus anterior; 14, fissura mediana anterior.

30

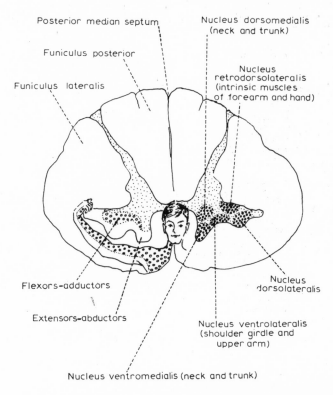

Posterior median septum

Funiculus posterior

Funiculus lateralis

Nucleus dorsomedialis
(neck and trunk)

Nucleus
retrodorsolateralis
(intrinsic muscles
of forearm and hand)

Flexors-adductors

Extensors-abductors

Nucleus
dorsolateralis

Nucleus ventrolateralis
(shoulder girdle and
upper arm)

Nucleus ventromedialis (neck and trunk)

Fig. 20. A diagrammatic representation of the distribution of columns of motor cells in the ventral horn in relation to the cells whose functions are concerned with flexion, extension, adduction or abduction. (After C.U. Ariëns Kappers.)

d. Intermediate grey (substantia grisea centralis and lateralis) contains cells with an internuncial or connective function acting as intermediaries between sensory and motor cells or between upper motor units of the cerebral cortex and lower motor cells of the spinal cord. It may include the inhibitory Renshaw cells.

3. Surrounding the inner grey nuclear zone is a mantle of white matter (Fig. 21), which is comprised of fibers which:
    a. Interconnect adjacent cord segments (fasciculus proprius) for interspinal reflexes.
    b. Project sensory information rostrally to higher centers.
        (i) Spinocerebellar tract (tractus spinocerebellaris) — unconscious proprioception (body position sense) to cerebellum.
        (ii) Anterolateral fasciculus (spinotectal, spinoreticular, spinothalamic tracts) — pathway for pain, temperature and light touch.

31

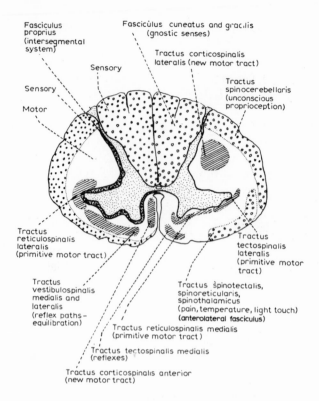

Fasciculus proprius (intersegmental system)

Fasciculus cuneatus and gracilis (gnostic senses)

Tractus corticospinalis lateralis (new motor tract)

Sensory

Tractus spinocerebellaris (unconscious proprioception)

Sensory

Motor

Tractus reticulospinalis lateralis (primitive motor tract)

Tractus tectospinalis lateralis (primitive motor tract)

Tractus vestibulospinalis medialis and lateralis (reflex paths – equilibration)

Tractus spinotectalis, spinoreticularis, spinothalamicus (pain, temperature, light touch) (anterolateral fasciculus)

Tractus reticulospinalis medialis (primitive motor tract)

Tractus tectospinalis medialis (reflexes)

Tractus corticospinalis anterior (new motor tract)

Fig. 21. A diagrammatic illustration of the various fiber bundles in the white matter of the spinal cord. Note that the intrinsic intersegmental fibers are closest to the grey matter, that the motor fibers are intermediate and the sensory projection fibers most peripheral (or dorsal).

(iii) Fasciculus cuneatus and gracilis (in dorsal funiculus) — conveys sensations of conscious proprioception, two-point discrimination, vibratory sense and stereognosis to the medulla where secondary neurons relay the information to the dorsal thalamus.

c. Conveys motor information from higher centers to appropriate cord levels for motor responses.

(i) Cortical control via the lateral and anterior corticospinal tracts (tractus corticospinalis lateralis and anterior).

(ii) Subcortical control via rubrospinal, vestibulospinal, tectospinal and reticulospinal tracts. The rubrospinal and reticulospinal systems provide for indirect corticospinal control of motor neurons of the spinal cord and cranial nerves.

d. A narrow commissural bundle (commissura alba) runs the entire length of the cord. It is in part associated with decussating fibers transmitting sensations of pain and temperature. It also contains fibers decussating from the anterior funiculus which terminate on cells of the ventral horn and have a motor function.

e. Note that the white matter of the ascending sensory projections tends to form the most peripheral group of fibers in the cord (and of the dorsal funiculus) and to be laminated into sacral (S), lumbar (L), thoracic (T) and cervical (C) units (Fig. 22).

4. Surface morphology. The spinal cord is separated into two halves by the posterior medial sulcus and the anterior medial fissure. Each half is further subdivided by the posterolateral sulcus and the anterolateral sulcus. This then creates a ventral (anterior), lateral and a posterior (dorsal) funiculus as gross subdivisions of white matter. The dorsal (posterior) funiculus is further subdivided in the upper thoracic and cervical regions into a fasciculus gracilis and a fasciculus cuneatus by the posterior intermediate sulcus.

a. The cord may be further noted to have two enlargements — cervical and lumbosacral, which correspond to the levels of origin of the brachial and lumbosacral plexuses.

B. Myelencephalon (medulla oblongata). Extends from its junction with the spinal cord at the foramen magnum rostrally to the pons from which it is separated by the bulbopontine sulcus ventrally and the striae medullares dorsally. The separation of the spinal cord from the medulla can be denoted on the ventral surface by the decussation of the pyramids. Note the acoustic tubercle (tuberculum acusticum) at the lateral aspect of the striae medullares.

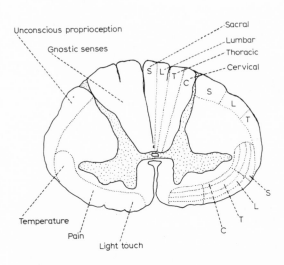

Fig. 22. This diagram demonstrates that there is a lamination in the pattern of organization of the ascending sensory projection systems. S, sacral; L, lumbar; T, thoracic; C, cervical.

33

1. Contains nuclear centers for several cranial nerves.

a. Hypoglossal nerve (XII) — motor innervation of tongue.

b. Vagus nerve (X) — motor innervation of pharyngeal constrictor muscles and muscles of speech and the parasympathetic components to the heart, lungs and abdominal viscera. It also contains an important sensory component related to cardiac and respiratory reflex regulation.

c. Glossopharyngeal nerve (IX) — innervation of the stylopharyngeal muscle and a visceral component associated with taste and general visceral sensations from the posterior tongue and oral nasal cavity plus motor innervation of the parotid gland.

d. Vestibulocochlear nerve (VIII) — for auditory and vestibular functions.

e. Trigeminal nerve (V) — a descending component associated with pain, temperature and light touch from the face.

2. There are, in addition, various reticular nuclear regions associated with cardiovascular, respiratory and emetic reflexes, as well as the propagation of impulses associated with some reflex control of spinal motor activity. Specific nuclear groups are the nucleus gigantocellularis (projects caudally to the spinal cord and rostrally to higher centers including the thalamus), ventrolateral nucleus (projects to the cerebellum) and the dorsolateral reticular nucleus which projects to cranial nerve nuclei.

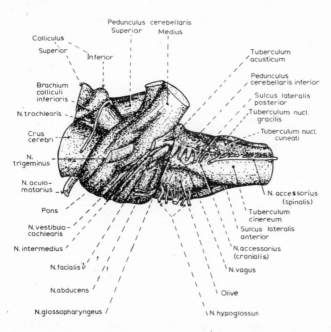

Fig. 23. The lateral aspect of the brain stem showing the medulla, pons and mesencephalon.

34

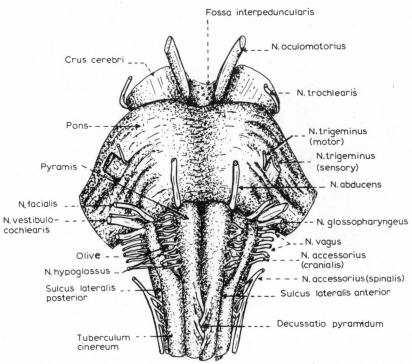

Fossa interpeduncularis

N. oculomotorius

Crus cerebri

N. trochlearis

Pons

N. trigeminus (motor)

N. trigeminus (sensory)

Pyramis

N. abducens

N. facialis

N. vestibulo-cochlearis

N. glossopharyngeus

N. vagus

Olive

N. accessorius (cranialis)

N. hypoglossus

N. accessorius (spinalis)

Sulcus lateralis posterior

Sulcus lateralis anterior

Decussatio pyramidum

Tuberculum cinereum

Fig. 24. The ventral aspect of the brain stem, showing the medulla, pons and mesencephalon.

3. Various sensory components for fine sensations of a discriminatory nature are relayed to higher levels by the dorsocaudal medullary nuclei (cuneatus and gracilis).

4. Various fiber bundles run through the medulla.
   a. Medial lemniscus — transmits fine discriminatory sensation to thalamus.
   b. Medial longitudinal fasciculus — associated with vestibular input and integrates cranial nerve activity.
   c. Tectospinal tract — fibers arising from superior colliculus involved in somatic, auditory and visual reflexes.

5. Motor fiber components arising from the cerebral cortex pass along the inferior margin (pyramids).

6. Surface markings unrelated to the ventricular floor (Figs 23 and 24).
   a. Protuberances. From posterior to anterior: clava (tuberculum gracilis), tuberculum cuneatum, inferior cerebellar peduncle (restiform body), trigeminal eminence (tuberculum cinereum), olive, pyramis (pyramid) and the decussation of the pyramids (decussatio pyramidum).

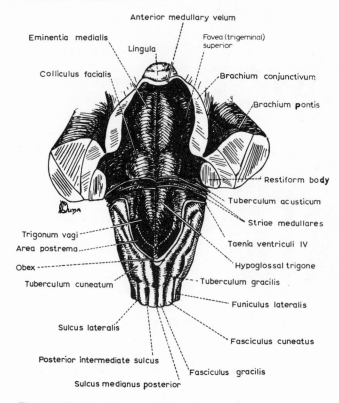

Anterior medullary velum

Eminentia medialis

Fovea (trigeminal) superior

Lingula

Colliculus facialis

Brachium conjunctivum

Brachium pontis

Restiform body

Tuberculum acusticum

Striae medullares

Trigonum vagi

Taenia ventriculi IV

Area postrema

Obex

Hypoglossal trigone

Tuberculum cuneatum

Tuberculum gracilis

Funiculus lateralis

Sulcus lateralis

Fasciculus cuneatus

Posterior intermediate sulcus

Fasciculus gracilis

Sulcus medianus posterior

Fig. 25. The dorsal aspect of the brain stem, showing the medullary and pontine portions of the floor of the fourth ventricle. Note the three peduncles of the cerebellum in relation to the lateral aspect of the ventricle: restiform body (inferior peduncle); brachium pontis (middle peduncle); and brachium conjunctivum (superior peduncle).

     b. Sulci: posteromedial sulcus, posterior intermediate sulcus, preolivary sulcus and postolivary sulcus (continuous with the anterolateral sulcus) and the anterior median fissure.

     c. Note the exiting or entering fibers of the various cranial nerves.

     7. Fourth ventricular surface (Fig. 25): posteromedial sulcus, hypoglossal trigone, sulcus limitans, inferior or vagal fovea (vagal trigone), obex, posterior half of vestibular trigone, striae medullares (separates pontine fourth ventricular floor from that of medulla).

C. Metencephalon (pons and cerebellum). Extends rostrally from the bulbo-pontine sulcus to the isthmus rhombencephali (the line of junction between the primitive hind- and midbrain vesicles). Is just caudal to the tectal or collicular plate of the mesencephalon.

1. Pons contains two primary units.

a. Pons basilaris (basal pons) — the large bulbous outgrowth at the inferior aspect which contains the large motor fiber bundles which arise in the cerebral cortex and project to the lower levels. These are longitudinally directed. There are also transverse running fibers arising from cells in the pons which relay information arising from the cerebral motor cortex to the contralateral cerebellar cortex via the middle cerebellar peduncle.

b. Pontine tegmentum. This is a direct continuation of the core of cells forming the medulla. It contains reticular nuclei whose fibers project either caudally, rostrally or to the adjacent nuclear structures. These nuclei also seem to be involved with various autonomic reflexes. There are in addition certain cranial nerve nuclei.

(i) Abducens nerve (VI) — for motor innervation of the external rotating muscle of the eye.

(ii) Facial nerve (VII) — for motor innervation of the facial musculature plus some autonomic innervation of visceral structures (glands) of the oral-nasal pharynx and of the submaxillary and lacrimal glands. There are, in addition, afferent fiber connections for taste from the anterior two-thirds of the tongue which terminate in a sensory nucleus.

(iii) The rostral portion of the medial vestibular nucleus and the superior vestibular nucleus (vestibular division of VIIIth nerve).

(iv) The superior olive. A nucleus associated with auditory function.

(v) Trigeminal nerve (V). The primary sensory nucleus for discriminative sensations and the motor nucleus for the muscles of mastication.

(vi) Fiber bundles passing through the tegmentum include the medial lemniscus, medial longitudinal fasciculus, the tectospinal tract and the central tegmental tract. The latter contains fibers arising in the central grey matter of the midbrain which terminates in the inferior olivary nucleus. Other fibers passing through the tract to terminate in the olive arise from the red nucleus. Another prominent fiber bundle which literally commences at the pontomedullary junction is the lateral lemniscus (auditory relay).

c. The ventral surface pontine morphology (see Figs 23 and 24). The basal pons is the large bulbous outgrowth from the anterior surface; the brachium pontis (middle cerebellar peduncle) projects posterolaterally from the basal pons. The point of separation between the pons and its brachia is the site of entrance for the fibers of the trigeminal nerve.

d. The dorsal ventricular pontine surface (Fig. 25) is divided into a medial eminence and a lateral portion by the sulcus limitans and superior or trigeminal fovea. The posteromedial sulcus continues rostrally from the region of the medulla. The caudal aspect of the medial eminence is enlarged to form the facial colliculus by the underlying abducens nucleus and genu of the facial nerve. The rostral portion of the vestibular trigone extends from the striae medullares to the superior fovea rostrally and laterally from the sulcus limitans to the acoustic tubercle in the lateral foramen of Luschka (apertura lateralis ventriculi quarti) of the fourth ventricle.

e. Caudally the pons is separated from the medulla by a circular sulcus running from one lateral foramen to the other in a ventral direction. This is the pontomedullary or bulbopontine sulcus. The region of the lateral foramen (of Luschka) is at the point of exit of the VIIth and VIIIth cranial nerves and is often referred to as the bulbopontine angle.

f. Rostrally the pons ends just caudal to the inferior colliculus dorsally and at the rostral margin of the basal pons ventrally. This line of demarcation is equivalent embryologically to the isthmus rhombencephali.

2. Cerebellum (Figs 26—28). This large multifoliated structure sits astride the brain stem oriented in a posterior or dorsal direction, being connected to the brain stem by three pairs of peduncles.

a. Inferior cerebellar peduncle (restiform body) passes up from the dorsum of the medulla into the cerebellum, conveying sensory information arising from the spinal cord relative to body position and from subcortical centers in relation to associated motor functions (via a relay through the inferior olivary nucleus).

b. Middle cerebellar peduncle (brachium pontis) relays information

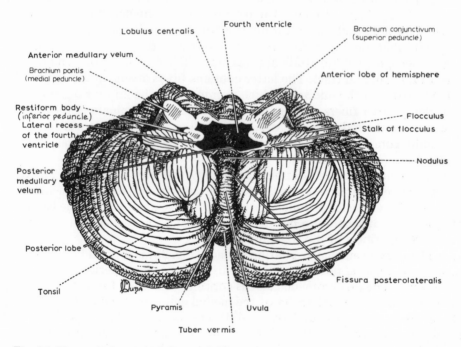

Fig. 26. The ventral aspect of the cerebellum.

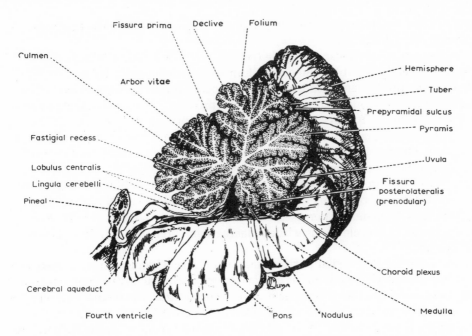

Fig. 27. The midsagittal plane through the brain stem illustrating the major units of the cerebellar vermis.

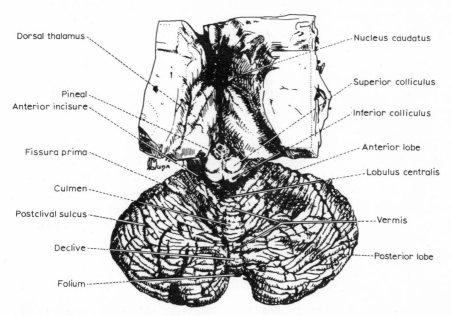

Fig. 28. The dorsal aspect of the cerebellum and brain stem as it continues rostrally with the diencephalon (dorsal thalamus).

39

arising originally from cerebral cortical areas. These fibers arise in the pons basilaris.

c. Superior cerebellar peduncle (brachium conjunctivum). This is the efferent projection limb of the cerebellum which relays the cerebellar influence via the thalamus to the cerebral motor and premotor cortex. Cerebellar connections with the red nucleus provide for a cerebellorubrospinal pathway, as well as for a cerebellorubrothalamic projection.

(i) This is accomplished by a cerebellar cortical projection to the deep cerebellar nuclei (dentate, globose and emboliform) which contain the final efferent cells for the cerebellar projection.

(ii) The cerebellum is usually considered to play a role in coordinating the actions of opposing muscle groups and in regulating the tonus of all muscles. In general, increased cerebellar output is associated with a decrease in muscle tonus while a decrease in cerebellar activity increases tonus.

d. Vermis — the medial portion between the two hemispheres. It arises early in embryonic development and is associated with truncal posture and coordination. In subserving these functions it may be noted that the medial vermian position is associated with truncal musculature; that the adjacent portion of the hemisphere is associated with the proximal part of the appendages and the most lateral part of the hemisphere with the distal portions of the extremities.

e. Flocculus. There are two flocculi, one overhanging each lateral foramen. They are very primitive phylogenetically and associated with equilibratory responses. Each is connected by a double-armed peduncle to the vestibular area in the pontine tegmentum and medulla and to the fastigial nuclei of the cerebellum.

f. Deep nuclei: dentate, emboliform, globose and fastigial. These are the relay nuclei which transmit cortical output arising from Purkinje cells to supra- and subcerebellar levels in the neuraxis. The fastigial nucleus is primarily associated with the vestibular system.

D. Mesencephalon (midbrain). The midbrain contains both ascending sensory and descending motor fiber components, reflex centers for auditory (inferior colliculus), somatic and visual response (superior colliculus) to the periphery, cranial nerve motor nuclei for extraocular muscles (oculomotor, III; and trochlear, IV), reticular nuclei, relay nuclei for cerebellar projections to the spinal cord (red nucleus and reticular nuclei) and an important subcortical nucleus (substantia nigra) concerned with associative motor functions. It is comprised of three fundamental units.

1. Tectum — superior and inferior colliculus.

2. Tegmentum — the deep nuclear part containing the cranial nerve nuclei, red nucleus, reticular nuclei and ascending somatic sensory and auditory pathways.

40

a. The fiber bundles of the medial lemniscus, medial longitudinal fasciculus, tectospinal tract and central tegmental fasciculus are also to be observed in the midbrain tegmentum. In addition, there are the decussating fiber bundles of the superior cerebellar peduncle as well as the ascending fibers of the auditory fiber projection system, the lateral lemniscus.

3. Pes pedunculi (crus cerebri), contains the descending corticobulbar and corticospinal motor units in conjunction with a corticopontine projection. This forms a large fiber bundle at the anterior (ventral) portion of the midbrain.
   a. Substantia nigra. A black to dark-brown pigmented nucleus intermediate in position between the pes pedunculi and the tegmentum which is related to the maintenance of such associative motor acts as arm swinging, quadrapedal progression and the facial expressions associated with speech.

4. Brachia of the midbrain.
   a. Brachium of the superior colliculus extends to the colliculus from the lateral geniculate body. Important in the light and accommodation reflexes.
   b. Brachium of the inferior colliculus extends from the colliculus to the medial geniculate body. Important in the relay of auditory sensations to higher levels.

E. Diencephalon. This is an egg-shaped structure which is essentially in the middle of the forebrain area (in the core of the cerebral hemisphere). Fig. 29 shows the part known as the dorsal thalamus and metathalamus. Ventral to this is a region known as the hypothalamus; also ventral and somewhat caudal is the subthalamus. The epithalamus (pineal and habenular trigones) is placed dorsomedially in the caudal region of the dorsal thalamus. The diencephalon extends from the lamina terminalis of the embryonic brain caudally to its junction with the midbrain in the region of the posterior commissure. The anterior commissure may also be considered a rostral marker. The two halves are separated from each other medially by the third ventricle (ventriculus tertius), although they are often joined by a small cellular bridge, the massa intermedia (adhesio interthalamica), which extends across the ventricle. Laterally the diencephalon is bounded by the internal capsule. The diencephalon is in a sense the "tween" brain, being between the midbrain (mesencephalon) and the forebrain structures of the cerebral hemisphere and the deep nuclei (basal ganglia) of the hemisphere. Being in this intermediate position, some of the diencephalic components will serve a specific intermediary role.

1. Non-specific relay nuclei.
   a. These are the nuclei of the internal and external medullary laminae, centrum medianum, and midline nuclei. They relay afferent information

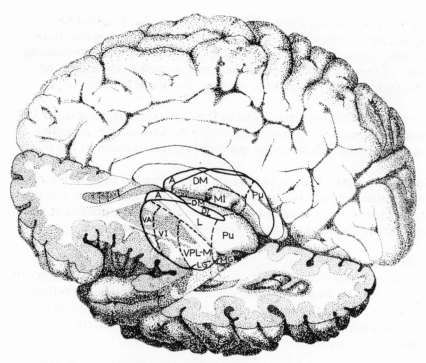

Fig. 29. A diagrammatic representation of the thalamus in its relative position in relation to the cerebral hemispheres. Note the essential central location. The approximate positions of the major dorsal thalamic nuclei are also indicated. A, anterior nucleus; DL, dorsolateral nucleus; DM, dorsomedial nucleus; L, posterolateral nucleus; Pu, pulvinar; VA, ventro-anterior nucleus; VI, ventrointermediate or -lateral nucleus; VPL-M, ventroposteromedial and -lateral nuclei. The nuclei of the metathalamus are also indicated: LG, lateral geniculate body and MG, medial geniculate body.

relative to light touch, pain and temperature to the limbic cortex via the internal capsule without any specificity of projection.

2. Specific projection nuclei.

a. These are the ventroposterolateral and medial nuclei which relay two-point discrimination, vibratory sense, conscious proprioception and stereo-gnosis from the body and face. Relays with a highly specific topographic pattern to areas 3, 1 and 2 of the sensory cortex via the internal capsule. There are also some terminals in the motor cortex, area 4.

b. The ventrolateral and ventral anterior nuclei relay cerebellar and basal nuclear output to the motor and premotor cortex. Fibers from both of these nuclei reach the cortex via the internal capsule. The anterior nucleus is in the limbic circuit, relaying hippocampal output from the mammillary bodies to area 24 of the gyrus cinguli via the internal capsule.

c. The medial geniculate body is a specific projection nucleus for audition to the superior transverse temporal gyrus, while the lateral geniculate body projects visual information to the calcarine cortex in the occipital lobe. The geniculate bodies project to the cortex via the sub- and retrolenticular portion of the internal capsule.

3. Associational nuclei.

a. The dorsomedial and posterolateral nuclei, and the pulvinar of the dorsal thalamus seem to have a role in integrating various regions of the cerebral cortex with each other. These nuclei also establish their cortical connections via the internal capsule. The dorsomedial nucleus and anterior thalamic nuclei are also connected to the frontal and temporal lobes via the thalamic peduncle.

4. Visceral nuclei. The hypothalamus is an important visceral center in the brain. It influences both sympathetic and parasympathetic systems. It contains regions associated with temperature regulation, feeding, satiety and thirst centers and regions concerned with cardiovascular regulation. Furthermore, it liberates hormones (vasopressin from the supraoptic nucleus, and oxytocin from the paraventricular nucleus, as well as the releasing factors now known to be important in regulating anterior pituitary function). It has connections with the basal nuclei (amygdala and globus pallidus), preoptic areas, septal areas and midbrain which make it important in reproductive and social behavior. The hypothalamus is associated with the rest of the CNS via numerous tract or fiber bundles.

a. Afferent fibers.

(i) Mammillary peduncle from dorsal and deep midbrain tegmental nuclei to mammillary bodies and lateral hypothalamus.

(ii) From periaqueductal grey.

(iii) Fornix from the hippocampus.

(iv) Medial forebrain bundle from frontal lobe and preoptic area.

b. Efferent fibers.

(i) Mammillothalamic tract to anterior nucleus of thalamus.

(ii) Projections via the dorsal longitudinal fasciculus to autonomic centers (caudally located).

(iii) Mammillotegmental tract to midbrain.

(iv) Hypothalamohypophyseal tract from the supraoptic paraventricular nuclei to the neurohypophysis.

(v) Hypothalamohypophyseal portal system. This is a vascular link between the hypothalamus and the adenohypophysis for transmission of the releasing factors concerned with pituitary synthesis or release of trophic hormones.

(vi) The optic tracts (tractus opticus) are often listed anatomically as part of the hypothalamus. Actually, they are not true nerves but brain tracts terminating primarily in the lateral geniculate bodies. The true optic nerves are within the retina. Functionally, the optic tracts would appear to have little direct relationship to the hypothalamus.

5. The pineal gland component of the epithalamus would appear to have some role in visceral activity in that it appears to secrete a hormone which retards sexual maturation.

6. Motor activity. The subthalamic nucleus is anatomically closely associated with the globus pallidus and would seem to be linked with the basal nuclei in influencing the function of the motor and premotor cortex.

F. Reticular formation. Throughout the brain stem (medulla through the midbrain) there are numerous ascending and descending nerve fiber bundles. There are also various special, well-delineated nuclear groups such as the cranial nerve nuclei, red nucleus or substantia nigra. Surrounding these nuclei is a meshwork of fibers and less well-delineated nuclear regions, which have a somewhat disordered appearance when stained with fiber stains. This meshwork is the reticular formation. It is not actually disorganized, however, and provides the nuclear and fiber substrate which plays a role in the function of cardiovascular and respiratory regulation, in emetic control, in the caudal relay for autonomic activation and for the integration of a number of spinal cord bulbar reflexes. Its anatomical organization is such that it may relay spinal cord sensory input to the thalamus and cortical (motor) information to various cranial nerve nuclei and to the spinal cord. The ascending relay function has been established as providing for an ascending reticular activation of the diencephalon and cerebral cortex. Some of the more prominent reticular nuclei (other than the red nucleus) are:

1. Medial reticular formation of the medulla (includes nucleus giganto-cellularis) — reticulospinal and supramedullary projections.

2. Dorsolateral reticular formation of the medulla — interacts with cranial nerve nuclei.

3. Ventrolateral reticular formation of medulla — projects afferent signals to cerebellum.

4. Ponto- and mesencephalic reticular formation areas have prominent rostral projections to the nonspecific projection nuclei of the thalamus as well as some descending projections into the cord.

G. Telencephalon. Divided into two general cellular regions separated from each other by white matter.

1. Cerebral cortex. The outer cellular layer of grey matter which is present in each lobe of the hemisphere.

a. Frontal lobe. Rostral to central sulcus and dorsal to lateral fissure. Has a prominent role in motor function.

b. Parietal lobe. Caudal to central sulcus and dorsal to lateral fissure. Separated from occipital lobe by an imaginary line. Has a significant role in somatic sensory perception.

c. Occipital lobe. Related to the back part of the brain caudal to the parietal lobe. Has a primary role in visual perception.

d. Temporal lobe. Inferior to the lateral fissure. Involved in relay of sensory information to the frontal lobe. Is the primary cortical site for auditory reception and is also significantly involved in memory.

(i) In the left hemisphere there is a half ring of cortex surrounding the lateral fissure which plays a role in language communication. It involves frontal lobe (motor communication) and the parietotemporal cortex where they are adjacent at the caudal and inferior margin of the lateral fissure (sensory perception in use of language).

e. Insula — a small island of cortex buried within the lips of the lateral fissure which seems to have a role in visceral sensory-motor activity.

2. Basal nuclei (ganglia). These are deep nuclei which are clearly associated with the motor cortex and which also possess reciprocal connections with the diencephalon and midbrain.

a. Caudate nucleus (head, body and tail). Lies along the margin of the lateral ventricle and is present in all parts except the posterior horn.

b. Lenticular nucleus. The putamen and globus pallidus which are found lateral to the internal capsule.

c. Amygdala. A small rounded nucleus at the rostral tip of the inferior horn of the lateral ventricle, just adjacent to the rostral inferior margin of the lenticular nucleus. Has close anatomical and functional associations with the hypothalamus and limbic system.

d. Claustrum. A thin lamina of cells interposed between the lenticular nucleus and the insula, enclosed by the external and extreme capsules.

3. White matter. Consists of myelinated nerve fibers which interconnect thalamus with cortex reciprocally, which project from the cortex to lower units such as cranial nerve and spinal cord motor cells and the pons (projection fibers), fibers which interconnect gyri of the same cortical side (long or short arcuate fibers), or which interconnect comparable areas of the two hemispheres (commissural fibers).

4. Olfactory brain. This part of the brain is composed of the medial and lateral olfactory striae which embrace the anterior perforated substance and the olfactory stalk and bulb. The stalk and bulb represent a projection of the

telencephalon which contains a fiber tract and associated nuclei along the tract. The olfactory striae are actually small gyri. The true olfactory nerves arise from within the olfactory mucosa, where the cell bodies are located. They penetrate the lamina cribrosa to reach the olfactory bulb. The cortex in the region of the limen insulae and the piriform cortex along the rostro-medial aspect of the temporal lobe are also associated with the olfactory portion of the brain.

5. Gyri and sulci. See Figs 30—32.

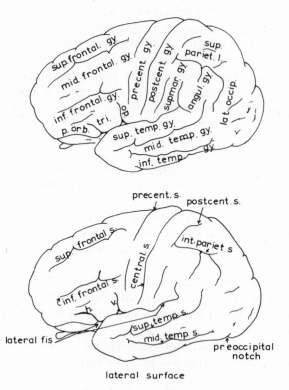

lateral surface

Fig. 30. A diagrammatic representation of the gyri and fissures as seen on the lateral surface of the cerebral hemisphere. gy., gyrus; inf. mid. and sup., inferior, middle and superior; s, sulcus; h., horizontal; v., vertical; p. orb., pars orbitalis; tri., pars triangularis; op., pars opercularis.

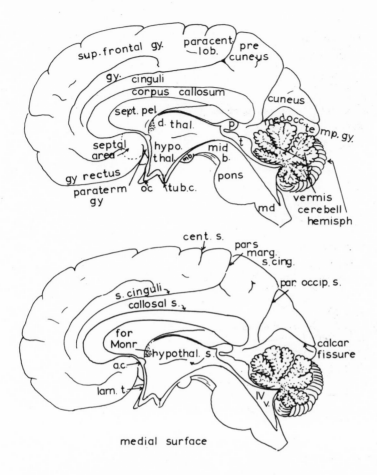

sup. frontal gy. paracent -lob. pre cuneus

gy. cinguli

corpus callosum cuneus

sept. pel d. thal. P med. occ. te mp. gy.

septal area hypo. thal. mid b. t

gy rectus paraterm gy oc tub.c. pons md vermis cerebell hemisph

cent. s.

pars marg. s. cing.

s. cinguli par. occip. s.

callosal s.

for Monr calcar fissure

a.c. hypothal. s.

lam. t. IV v.

medial surface

Fig. 31. A diagrammatic representation of the sulci and gyri on the midsagittal surface of the cerebral hemisphere. gy., gyrus; s., sulcus; mid b., midbrain; med. occ. temp. gy., medial occipital temporal gyrus; d. thal., dorsal thalamus; md, medulla; for Monr, foramen of Monro; a.c., anterior commissure; lam. t., lamina terminalis; oc, optic chiasm; mb, mammillary body; IV v., fourth ventricle.

47

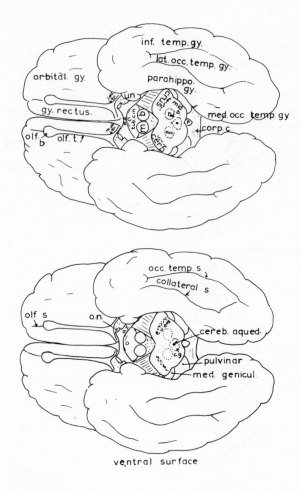

inf. temp. gy.
lat. occ. temp. gy.
orbital. gy.
parahippo.
gy.
un
gy. rectus.
med. occ. temp. gy
olf. b. olf. t.
corp. c

occ. temp. s.
collateral s.
olf s
o.n.
cereb. aqued.
pulvinar
med. genicul.

ventral surface

Fig. 32. The ventral surface of the cerebral hemisphere. gy., gyrus; s., sulcus; inf., inferior; lat., lateral; olf. b. and olf. t., olfactory bulb and tract; o.n., o.c. and o.t., optic nerve, chiasm and tract; tub. cin., tuber cinereum; mb, mammillary body; c.g., central grey; sub. n., substantia nigra; p, pineal; corp. c., corpus callosum.

Chapter 3

THE FUNCTIONAL UNIT: THE NEURON

While there is a considerable body of evidence which implies that neurons function metabolically in relation to the glial cells which surround them (forming neuroglial functional units), it is easier to examine these two cell types independently, particularly in a discussion of morphology.

The neuron is a highly differentiated cell whose role appears to be directed toward the propagation of an impulse by a combination of electrical and chemical processes. Associated with this phenomenon is the tacit assumption that neurons are in some way involved in learning and memory storage. This may involve neurons in various related groups which interact with each other as a result of being stimulated by an appropriate signal, and it may further involve the storage of information within some membrane unit of the neuron in the form of macromolecules. The neuron may be further differentiated from other cell types in that it is essentially unable to undergo cell division in the postnatal period. Thus, the neurons with which one is born essentially constitute the total number one is ever to have. This excepts observations from a number of workers that small neurons of the granule cell variety may undergo division in the cerebellar and hippocampal cortex for appreciable periods after birth. One may further note that the neuron population in man is not constant and that neurons are lost in extreme old age. However, reliable data for areas other than cortex are not generally available.

As examined by light or electron microscopy, the neuron is generally characterized by having a relatively large, pale-staining nucleus and prominent nucleolus. Large clumps of basophilic material described initially by Nissl are observed to abound in neurons and to vary considerably from one neuronal type to another and to be readily altered by activity and pathological processes. These Nissl granules represent the coalescence of RNA and protein as ribosomes on the endoplasmic reticulum, as seen in other cells. In general, therefore, it will be observed that neurons contain the same general intracellular constituents as do other mature cell forms (Fig. 33). Neurons also have extracellular processes. Some (dendrites) are receptive, while others (axons) are projective. Further, axons assume a specific relation with various supportive cells (Schwann cells in the peripheral nervous system and oligodendroglial cells in the CNS), in which the supportive cells provide a covering of myelin around many axons. There are finally the terminal endings of axons which transmit a signal initiated in one neuron to the next neuron or effector cell. There are also various intracellular inclusions such as lipofuscin or

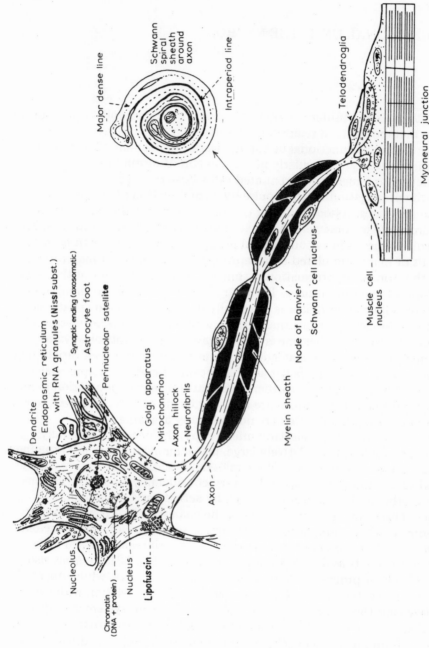

Nucleolus

Chromatin
(DNA + protein)

Nucleus

Lipofuscin

Dendrite

Endoplasmic reticulum
with RNA granules (Nissl subst.)

Synaptic ending (axosomatic)

Astrocyte foot

Perinucleolar satellite

Golgi apparatus

Mitochondrion

Axon hillock

Neurofibrils

Axon

Myelin sheath

Node of Ranvier

Schwann cell nucleus

Major dense line

Schwann
spiral
sheath
around
axon

Intraperiod line

Telodendroglia

Muscle cell
nucleus

Myoneural junction

Fig. 33. A diagrammatic representation of a multipolar neuron showing the major organelles, processes and termination at a myoneural junction. Note that the myelin sheath is not a solid mass of lipid wrapped around an axon, but a spiral of Schwann cell cytoplasmic membranes wound around the axon. The telodendroglia overlying the neuro-muscular endplate is a type of modified glial cell. Note that the various organelles are not drawn to scale.

melanin pigments. Lipofuscin and accumulations of oddly shaped neuro-fibrillar elements increase with age.

A. The cell membrane. This is comparable to that of all cells having two electron-dense layers separated by a relatively structureless inner zone forming a membrane with a total thickness of 70—80Å. These two layers differ slightly morphologically in that the inner lamina is slightly thicker. The middle electron-lucent layer is 25—30Å wide. This membrane is continuous and clearly defines the boundary of the cell. Local modifications of the membrane occur at synaptic and adhesive junctions.

B. Typically, neurons have large, relatively pale-staining nuclei, which, how-ever, have virtually as much DNA as do liver, pancreatic, muscle or kidney cells (2.3×10^{-12} g). There are, however, neurons which are tetraploid or occasionally octaploid (Purkinje cells of the cerebellar cortex) which have more DNA. The nucleus is usually round and located in the center of the cell. The thin nuclear membrane is often separated from other cell organelles by a clear halo of structureless cytoplasm. The nucleus, as in other cell types, has been observed to rotate. The karyoplasm is generally clear, but in smaller neurons with smaller nuclei, wherein the amount of DNA is the same, it may be as dense as that of lymphocytes. Not all nuclei are symmetrical, being irregularly creased or folded. These creases or folds are generally filled with a basophilic cytoplasm resembling Nissl substance or as free ribosomes.

1. The nuclear membrane consists of two laminae each about 70Å thick which are separated by a space of varying width. The inner membrane is usually smooth, while the outer membrane tends to be somewhat folded and irregular. The intervening space or nuclear cistern is in many places continuous with the endoplasmic reticulum (which has been observed to arise from the outer nuclear membrane).

a. There are numerous pores in the nuclear membrane which may provide for some degree of interaction between components of the karyo-plasm and cytoplasm. These pores appear to be loosely closed by some form of diaphragm. Thus, these are not "open" pores, but perhaps only regions of attenuation of the nuclear membrane.

b. The chromatin of the nucleus is in an extended form in fine strands.

c. The nucleolus appears as a dense basophilic structure which under the electron microscope appears to consist of dense granules and very fine filaments. This is presumably mostly RNA or ribonuclear protein. DNA is also present. In the newborn or in regenerating neurons it clumps at opposite poles. In normal mature neurons it is distributed throughout the nucleolus and not revealed by standard staining procedures. A third component seen in other cell types consists of chromatin. This is usually seen in neurons from females where the heterochromatic X chromosome is attached to the nucleolar surface as the nucleolar satellite.

d. Filaments clumped in bundles have been reported in the nuclei of a number of neurons. Some of these filaments appear to interact with each other to form a crystalline lattice. Further, in cells of the lateral vestibular nucleus these filaments have been observed with microtubules.

C. Cytoplasmic constituents.

1. Nissl substance. The very basophilic material which appears in chunks or blocks, as seen by light microscopy, appears on electron microscopy as a complex of ribosomes studding the endoplasmic reticulum. Its appearance varies with cell type from the large angular blocks in motor cells to small dust-like particles in small ganglion cells. In larger granule cells it is arranged in small particles concentrated at the periphery of the perikaryon. Further, there are many intermediate forms. Many investigators have demonstrated that the appearance of the Nissl material varies with the degree of cell activity (accumulates in large amounts in nonactive cells and is relatively scarce in very active neurons). It undergoes dissolution in a damaged or dying neuron undergoing the process of chromatolysis. It is customarily found only in the soma and dendrites, while neither the axon nor the axon hillock contain RNA related to endoplasmic reticulum. However, RNA is found in axons either as free ribosomes or in a soluble form. The RNA and free ribosomes of neurons, as elsewhere, play a significant role in protein synthesis.

2. Golgi apparatus. This is a special configuration of agranular endoplasmic reticulum which by electron microscopy is seen to consist of a complex of broad, flattened cisternae which appear to be piled in stacks with very little intervening space. Clusters of small vesicles are also associated with this grouping. Metal impregnation stains and light microscopy show a cell-wide Golgi system. This organelle was first described in neurons. Evidence from a number of fields links the Golgi apparatus to synthetic mechanisms of the cell.

a. The Golgi apparatus, endoplasmic reticulum and the lysosomes in neurons have been linked together as a single system called the GERL system by Novikoff *et al.*

3. Multivesicular bodies. These are small (0.5μm) spherical structures, limited by a unit membrane, which contain a varying number of small vesicles. Although found throughout the neuron and its processes, they are most commonly found in association with the Golgi apparatus. Many workers believe them to be related to lysosomes.

4. Lysosomes. These are the so-called dark bodies previously reported from studies using light microscopy. They contain large amounts of acid phosphatase

and other hydrolytic enzymes such as ribonuclease.

5. Lipofuscin granules. These are greenish yellow granules which increase in certain neurons with age, often obscuring other organelles. It is now believed that they may be derived from lysosomes.

6. Microtubules and neurofilaments. These are conspicuous tubular and filamentous structures found throughout the soma and processes of neurons and are of unknown function.

7. Cilia and centrioles. Cilia have been observed arising from a number of neuronal types in a number of species. They differ from cilia in general, however, in that they contain only the nine longitudinal doublets of microtubules and lack the central core pair of microtubules. They are apparently motionless. Retinal rods and cones are also ciliary derivatives. The basal bodies of neural cilia resemble those of other cells and consist of nine evenly spaced triplets of microtubules arranged longitudinally to form a cylinder. Thin rootlets may then radiate out into the surrounding cytoplasm. The neural cilium may also have a centriole suspended in the cytoplasm at right-angles below the basal body.

8. Laminated and fibrillary inclusions. These are made up of regularly spaced sheets of microtubules embedded in a dense matrix, frequently with some swirling.

9. Secretory products. These are seen by both light and electron microscopy in cells of the supraoptic and paraventricular nuclei as small granules which may coalesce into droplets. These droplets consist of a protein called neurophysin which is associated with the active hormones vasopressin and oxytocin.

10. Pigments other than lipofuscin occur in neurons such as the black or brown melanin-like pigments of the cells of the substantia nigra and locus ceruleus. Cells of the substantia nigra contain dopamine, a transmitter associated with Parkinsonism.

11. Mitochondria. These small organelles which consist of an outer membranous envelope and an inner membrane folded into cristae are found in all parts of a neuron. They are involved in aerobic and anaerobic glycolysis. In the synaptic terminals of axons they appear to have a role in the metabolism of transmitter substances. Further, in the neonatal brain, thyroid hormone stimulates mitochondrial-mediated protein synthesis.

12. Synaptic apparatus. This consists of a very special adaptation of the neuronal membrane at its functional contact with the membrane of either

the next neuron or some other effector cell. The membranes are thicker than elsewhere and there may be some form of matrix material between the opposing cells. The distance at the synaptic cleft which separates the two cells is 150—200Å or slightly less than the intercellular space at nonsynaptic sites. Synaptic vesicles 300—400Å in diameter are abundant in the presynaptic region. They may be oval or round and may or may not contain an electron-dense material. The clear vesicles are cholinergic and the dense-appearing vesicles are apparently aminergic (i.e. norepinephrine). Neurons of the nucleus of the median raphe of the mesencephalon synthesize serotonin, which may be seen by fluorescence microscopy in the cell body and processes. It presumably also becomes enclosed in synaptic vesicles. Further, there are, in the postsynaptic junctional units of other neurons, various types of subsynaptic organelles which appear as dense webs or series of processes projecting into the cell. Another characteristic of the synaptic terminal is the large number of mitochondria in the presynaptic component.

a. Types of synapse. There are basically three types of synapse in the CNS: axo-dendritic, axo-somatic, and axo-axonal. There have also been described what may be termed dendrodendritic synapses. The axo-somatic type of junction lacks a subsynaptic organelle. There are also what has been termed tight junctions or electrical synapses wherein the synaptic cleft is obliterated and the cell membranes fuse together (in fishes and frogs).

b. Some synapses occur in a rather structured way, surrounded by numerous astrocytic processes which have been considered as isolating the unit from other influences. The astrocytes at synaptic junctions also seem important at cholinergic junctions, since they are rich in cholinesterase. Isolated synaptosomes are also rich in cholinesterase.

D. Neuronal processes. There are two fundamental types: axons and dendrites.

1. Axons are the efferent processes of neurons. They may give off side branches, collateral or recurrent processes. Other than this, however, the surface membranes of the axons have no additional types of side process. By electron microscopy the axon has been observed to contain neurofibrils and tubules, mitochondria and ribosomes. Synaptic vesicles are then finally observed at the terminal end. Synaptic vesicles have also been observed along the course of small unmyelinated axonal processes. This occurs frequently in the autonomic system. These axons pass over a number of units which will be innervated en passant. Vesicles occur at each of the sites where the axon makes contact with a structure to be innervated. Axons within the CNS will have a myelin sheath formed by processes arising from oligodendroglial cells. Axons of the peripheral nervous system will also be covered by myelin but, in this instance, it will be formed by Schwann cells. There are also unmyelinated axons in the CNS.

a. Axons of the autonomic nervous system postganglionic units appear virtually unmyelinated. However, each fiber will be surrounded by a single Schwann cell lamella.

b. Axoplasmic flow refers to the concept that the axoplasm is in a dynamic state, being formed largely in the neuronal soma from whence it flows out into the axon, serving to provide for its metabolic maintenance. Weiss was amongst the first contributors to the concept of axoplasmic flow. Since his observations it has been observed to be important in the movement of neurosecretory products down the axon toward the terminals in the posterior pituitary gland.

The observation that proteins move along the axon toward its terminal end raises questions relative to the fate of such protein. While this is still uncertain, it would appear that some is degraded, since there are endo- and exopeptidases in the nerve fibers. Furthermore, mitochondria and their membrane components have been demonstrated to possess sufficient proteolytic activity to account for known rates of neuronal protein turnover.

Axoplasmic flow has been observed to consist of two principle components. There is a fast component which flows at a rate of 400 mm per day in the cat and dog and a slow component which flows at a rate of less than 100 mm per day. With labelling studies with tritiated amino acids it has been shown that the fast component contains labelled free amino acids, polypeptides and soluble protein. The slow component consists primarily of soluble protein. The soluble protein has been further characterized into two categories, one with a molecular weight of 68 000 and the other with a molecular weight of 450 000. Although axoplasmic flow may provide the main source of materials for metabolic maintenance of the axon, there is evidence demonstrating that protein synthesis also occurs along the length of the axon which is not dependent on a supply of protein from the soma. Finally, it may be noted that axoplasmic flow is energy dependent in its movement down the axon. It may also be bidirectional. In the processes of the dorsal root ganglion cell, axoplasmic flow has been observed in both the afferent and efferent components. Since both have essentially the structure of an axon, being myelinated, it is not yet possible to state whether or not such flow occurs in other afferent (dendritic) processes which lack myelin.

2. Dendrites are the afferent processes of CNS neurons and are unmyelinated. When studied by the Golgi-Cox technique, they appear to be covered with numerous short side branches or spines. These may be very short or up to a micron or so in length. The spines are a preferred site of synaptic contact (axo-spinous synapse). Electron microscopy reveals that dendrites contain neurotubules and fibrils, mitochondria and rough endoplasmic reticulum. Synaptic vesicles are not seen.

E. Types of neurons. There are basically three types of neurons: unipolar, bipolar and multipolar.

1. Unipolar neurons are characteristically found only in sensory ganglia and have a round or oval shape. While in other neurons the efferent or axonal component is the myelinated fiber, with sensory neurons both the afferent and efferent limbs are coated with myelin. All unipolar neurons in ganglia are further characterized by having a double-layered capsule.

a. Satellite cells (modified glial units) form an inner, completely investing capsule. Like the ganglion cells, they are derived from the neural crest.

b. Fibroblastic cells form an outer capsule which becomes associated with the connective tissue of the ganglia.

c. The unipolar cells of the mesencephalic nucleus of the trigeminal nerve are the only unipolar cells within the CNS and are not encased in a sheath of satellite cells.

2. Bipolar cells are characteristically associated with the specialized receptor units of the nervous system.

a. The receptor cells of the olfactory epithelium.

b. The primary neurons of the vestibulocochlear nerve in the spiral ganglion of the ear and the ganglion of Scarpa of the vestibular apparatus (the cell bodies of these neurons are myelinated).

c. The bipolar relay cells of the retina.

3. Multipolar cells with a great many different types of morphological forms and size constitute the rest of the neuronal population. The name appended to these cells denotes either their general morphological shape, as in pyramidal, granule, fusiform or basket cell, or the name of the anatomist who first described them (Purkinje, cells of Martinotti and of Cajal). Some of these are illustrated in Fig. 34. As observed using the Golgi-Cox technique, axons are bare of short side processes while dendrites are generally covered by a great many short processes or spines (Fig. 35). The two pyramidal cells shown in Fig. 35 are taken from adjacent areas of the hippocampus and show the cell body in the stratum pyramidale with the dendrites projecting up into the outer layers which are deficient in neurons (comparable to the "molecular layer" of the cerebral cortex). The axon is seen projecting out into the white matter of the hippocampus, the alveus which leads into the fornix.

a. Postganglionic autonomic cells are encapsulated (like cells of the dorsal root ganglia) with a layer of satellite cells derived from the neural crest.

F. Myelinization. The myelin sheath begins a short distance from the cell

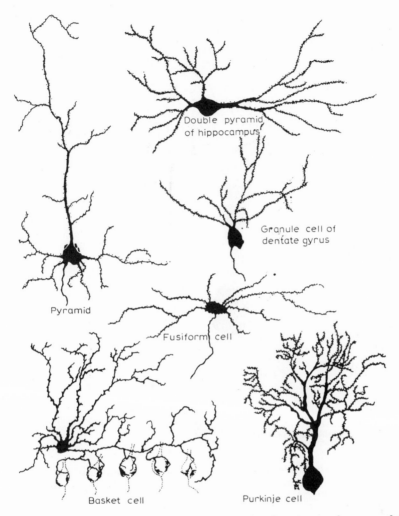

Fig. 34. A representation of the appearance of various types of neurons following one of the metal impregnation techniques. Note that these are all multipolar neurons, that the dendrites have numerous spines and that the axons consist of bare processes.

and stops just before the axon terminates at a synapse. Peripherally myelin is formed by the Schwann cells, while centrally it is formed by processes derived from the interfascicular oligodendroglia. The sheath is of varying thickness, semifluid in nature and contains protein, phospholipids, certain cerebrosides and fatty acids. The myelin sheath is interrupted at intervals along the fibers by the nodes of Ranvier. Branching of a neuron frequently occurs at these nodes. The axons narrow at the termination of the myelin around a fiber at a node and bulge slightly in the internodal region. In the

57

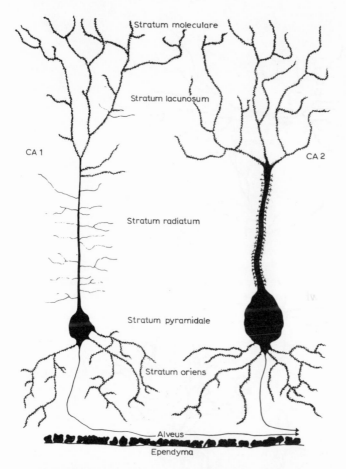

Fig. 35. A representation of two different pyramidal cell types in the cortex of the hippocampus illustrating differences in soma size and dendritic formation in different, but adjacent, regions (CA1 and CA2) as described by Cajal.

peripheral nervous system, finger-like processes of adjacent Schwann cells interdigitate with each other around the nodal zone, while in the CNS the nodal area is bare. Axo-axonal en passant synapses may occur at these sites. Axons may branch at these sites as well.

1. Peripheral myelin formation. As myelin first begins to form around a peripheral axon it appears as if the axon sinks into the cytoplasm of a Schwann cell, becoming surrounded by a layer of the cytomembrane of the Schwann cell, being suspended much like the intestine is in the mesentery. One portion of the Schwann cell process then begins to grow under the other, forming a sort of jelly roll which surrounds the axon until many

layers of processes have wrapped around the axon (may be up to 100). The cytoplasm of these processes becomes squeezed out, bringing the various layers of Schwann cell membranes together. The inner layers fuse together to form the major dense lines, while the outer surfaces of the membrane also fuse to form the intraperiod line. Cell membranes are really asymmetric, with the inner lamina being slightly thicker. This explains the fusion of the two inner laminae of the Schwann membrane giving rise to the major dense lines, while the fusion of the two thinner, outer laminae give rise to the thinner intraperiod line. The Schwann cell organelles then become concentrated around the nucleus and in small projecting processes in the nodal regions. This fusion results in a repeating series of light and dark lines as seen by electron microscopy and X-ray diffraction. As this rolling up of the axon occurs, each succeeding layer going from the innermost layer outward overlaps the preceding layer. There is a basement membrane surrounding each Schwann unit.

a. Schmidt-Lantermann clefts. These were originally believed to be breaks in the myelin sheath as seen by light microscopy. It now appears that they occur in regions where adjacent lamellae of the myelin sheath have come unstuck along the intraperiod line. Thus, these spaces should be continuous with the extracellular space. It further appears that they may be in a state of dynamic movement and may well, as earlier suggested, serve to facilitate transport of nutrients into the axon. This seems all the more plausible from recent studies which suggest that metabolic support of the axon need not be entirely dependent on axoplasmic flow and that there is some active protein synthesis which does occur along the length of an axon.

2. Central myelin formation. The interfascicular oligodendroglia have been observed by several electron microscopists to form the multilamellar sheaths of central myelin. In this instance each oligodendroglia may be involved in contributing processes to several adjacent axons. There are no basement membranes surrounding the central myelinated units.

3. Unmyelinated fibers. These are very thin axons (Remak fibers) of the postganglionic neurons of the autonomic system which are coated over with only a single layer of Schwann cell membrane instead of multiple series of Schwann membranes. They are also encountered in the CNS where they are coated by only a single layer of glial processes. Many axons of the CNS are completely devoid of glial investment.

4. Degree of myelinization. In general this depends on the axonal diameter. In tissue culture the critical diameter is $1\,\mu$m. Larger axons are always invested with myelin membranes with the largest fibers having the thickest sheaths.

G. Degeneration of axons. Inasmuch as the cell body is the primary trophic center of a neuron, damage to an axon which interferes with axoplasmic flow results in varying degrees of change in the distal segment, the severity being dependent on the extent of injury.

1. Wallerian degeneration. This refers to the changes occurring distal to the level of injury and begins almost immediately after a severe crush or cut. There is an accumulation of mitochondria at the nodes followed by breakdown of the axoplasm, neurofibrils and mitochondria. Within a few days the axon breaks up into fragments. The synaptic endings also show degenerative changes which are most readily appreciated by electron microscopy. Schwann cells undergo hypertrophy, hyperplasia and become mobile. They also become phagocytic and ingest the disintegrated myelin. These will then form what are literally tubes of Schwann cells with elaborately folded basement membranes, folded one inside the other within the endoneurium of the axon. Regenerating sprouts from the proximal segment of the nerve will grow into these tubes entering between the Schwann cell and its basement membrane. If no regrowth occurs, the Schwann tube will shrink and the walls will become thickened due to the increase of collagen in the endoneurium.

2. Retrograde degeneration. This refers to the changes in the proximal stump of a damaged nerve. If the injury is minor, as in a clean cut, only a few internodal segments may be involved. If there is considerable injury or inflammation, changes comparable to those seen in Wallerian degeneration may extend 2 to 3 cm up the proximal axonal segment.
a. There are also associated changes in the cell body. It becomes swollen, the Nissl material breaks down and the nucleus becomes shifted to the periphery of the cell (central chromatolysis with cloudy swelling). Electron microscopy studies suggest that the ribonucleoprotein of the Nissl substance is not so much lysed as dispersed. There are also ultrastructural changes in the mitochondria, Golgi apparatus and lysosomes. Further, histochemical and microchemical studies suggest that the total RNA (ribosomal, soluble and transport RNAs) is actually increased and that there is also an increase in nucleoprotein synthesis.
(i) Lesions near the cell body produce greater changes than those which are more distant. Further, neonatal cells seem more likely to fail to recover from the effects of axonal injury.
(ii) While changes seen by light microscopy seem to reach their maximal extent in 12 to 14 days, changes in RNA and protein synthesis associated with restoration of the cell appear to start much earlier.

3. Postsynaptic degeneration. This refers to the degeneration of neurons on which a degenerating fiber terminates. It is characteristically seen in the visual and cerebellar system. Thus, destruction of the axons in the central tegmental fasciculus leads to degeneration of the cells of the inferior olive on which they

60

terminate. This is followed by degeneration of the olivocerebellar fibers and finally degeneration of the cerebellar cortex. As yet there is no convincing explanation for this type of degeneration.

4. Regeneration. When a neuron survives injury, distinct changes seen by light microscopy are apparent within three weeks. New Nissl particles may be seen around the nucleus, the cell shrinks toward its normal size and the nucleus resumes its central position. However, full recovery may take three to six months, depending on the amount of axon to regrow. Numerous fine fibers emerge from the proximal stump of a severed axon as soon as ten hours after injury due to the pressure within the axon resulting from axoplasmic flow. These traverse the scar formed at the injury site and in about four days after lesioning enter the Schwann tube, being peripherally placed. Some will move more centrally later and become completely surrounded by the sheath cell membrane. While many axonal sprouts may enter a single Schwann tube, only one will persist and become remyelinated. This is usually the largest fiber. The other smaller sprouts are suppressed. Remyelinization of this fiber is then dependent on it re-establishing contact with the appropriate effector. (If it is the distal fiber of a sensory cell, the contact would be with an appropriate receptor.)

5. Central degeneration. This is essentially similar to peripheral degeneration except that it proceeds more slowly and the removal of neuronal debris by microglia and modified oligodendroglia is slower. Degeneration of large fibers proceeds faster than that observed in smaller fibers, but the degenerated products are resorbed more slowly.

a. Regeneration is known to occur in the CNS, but the attempts are usually abortive due to the failure of the axonal sprouts to penetrate the glial scars or the gaps between the severed stumps. Remyelinization of injured, but unsevered, nerves in the spinal cord has also been observed in cats by Bunge *et al.*, 1961.

Chapter 4

INTERNAL SUPPORTING ELEMENTS

The internal supporting cells of the nervous system are the glial cells, of which there are three general types: astrocytes, oligodendroglia and microglia. The term glia is most appropriate for these cells, since it means glue and the first two of these cell types do literally glue the CNS together. The macroglia (astrocytes and oligodendroglia) differ from neurons in that they have only one type of process, they do not form synapses and they retain the capacity to divide, particularly if there is damage to the CNS. Like the neurons, macroglia are derived from neural ectoderm. There is further an extensive gliogenesis which occurs postnatally and which is at least partly associated with myelin formation. However, numerous astrocytes and oligodendroglia are also formed whose function appears to be more related to biochemical support of neurons. Microglia, however, appear to be derived from mesoderm and are present in the CNS in large numbers only in association with disease or injury.

A. Astrocytes. These appear as star-shaped cells, when studied by the gold sublimate method of Cajal, with processes extending into the surrounding neuropil. Some of these processes will form end feet on capillary walls, others will have processes which extend to the surface of the brain to form expansions underlying the pia mater (glial limiting membrane), while others will form a similar limiting membrane beneath the ependymal cells. In addition, the protoplasmic astrocytes in the grey matter have numerous end feet in relation to the neuronal soma and dendrites. The astrocytes in white matter contain numerous fibrils and fine branching fibrous processes and thus are fibrous astrocytes. Astrocytes of the grey matter contain relatively few fibrils and, because of their many short branched processes, have been called proto-plasmic astrocytes. These too, however, will have some fibrils. In certain types of pathologic process (multiple sclerosis) the fibril content of astrocytes is greatly increased. These cells are very susceptible to edema as a result of hypoxia.

1. Fibrous astrocyte. These cells are lighter in appearance than other cells present in white matter as observed by electron microscopy. The nuclei are irregular and the nuclear envelope may be deeply folded. The nucleus has a fairly even intensity and a nucleolus may occasionally be seen. The most prominent cytoplasmic elements are the numerous fibrils (80—90Å) which, according to Bairati (1958), are formed of alpha-keratin. The usual organelles

are also present in the cytoplasm but are sparse as compared to other cells and, except for the mitochondria, are located around the nucleus. Numerous granules of glycogen are also present.

2. Protoplasmic astrocytes are found primarily in the grey matter, and like fibrous astrocytes are characterized by the presence of cytoplasmic fibrils, though there are fewer of them. Glycogen granules are also present. The nuclei appear relatively homogeneous and are more oval than those of fibrous astrocytes.

a. Fañanas cells of the cerebellar cortex and the Müller fibers of the retina appear to be modified forms of protoplasmic astrocytes.

3. Functions.

a. Structural support. They are interwoven amongst the neuronal processes and adherent to pia, providing for an outer sheath over the entire CNS. In the white matter the processes of fibrous astrocytes usually pass at right-angles to the nerve fibers and appear interwoven among them.

b. Repair. When there is structural damage to the CNS, the astrocytes form a type of scar in the degenerated area by proliferating and filling the area with their processes.

c. Transport. The arrangement of protoplasmic astrocytes with end feet surrounding the capillaries and with cytoplasmic processes which appear to bridge between the capillary and the soma and dendrites of the neuron has led to the concept that astrocytes may serve to facilitate transport of materials to neurons. This concept is further supported by the observation that pericapillary glia are rich in those enzymes which would appear suited for a transport role.

d. Isolation of receptive surfaces. Studies with the electron microscope indicate that astrocytes in certain areas show a patterned organization which appears designed to isolate the receptive surfaces of neurons, in conjunction with the synaptic endings, into compartments which would seem unlikely to be influenced by other elements (i.e. the terminals of basket cells around the axon hillock of the Purkinje cells of the cerebellar cortex are isolated from the surrounding tissue by many layers of astrocytic glial processes).

B. Oligodendroglia. The term was derived by del Rio-Hortega (1921) to describe cells with relatively few processes in neuronal material stained by metallic impregnation. Processes appear short as they project from a spherical or polygonal cell body. The nuclei also appear somewhat more chromophilic, smaller and more regular than those observed in astrocytes. The cytoplasm is also more chromophilic than in astrocytes. They are found in white matter, interspersed throughout the grey matter and as satellites around the neurons. They have few fibrils or glycogen particles, which further distinguishes them from astrocytes. Microtubules are numerous, however, making them resemble dendritic processes. Like astrocytes, oligodendroglia have no synaptic connections.

1. Functions.
a. Formation of myelin in the CNS white matter appears a major function for the interfascicular oligodendroglia. A single cell may contribute processes which enter into the formation of the myelin sheaths of a number of axons.

b. Nutritive support of neurons by the satellite cells. This form of symbiotic support is suggested by the studies of Hydén and co-workers who have observed an intimate association between perineuronal glia and the neuron in relation to respiratory enzyme function and RNA metabolism.

c. Phagocytosis of a dead neuron by its satellites has been claimed as an oligodendroglial function by various neuropathologists. There is in addition a glial proliferation around neuronal cell bodies whose axons are undergoing regeneration, presumably for enhanced metabolic support.

C. Microglia (rod cells, mesoglia) have elongated or triangular nuclei which stain intensely with basic dyes. There is a scanty cytoplasm from which arise short wavy processes which give off spine-like projections. They may be found in either white or grey matter, although they have been said to be more numerous in grey matter, where they are said to make up about 10% of the glial population. Other observers note that microglia are generally rarely seen in normal tissue. Microglia are said to be of mesodermal origin and to invade the CNS at the time of penetration by the vessels. Other observations suggest that they may be derived from the pericytes found in the walls of capillaries. By electron microscopy they appear as very electron-dense cells, filled with granules, with nuclei that have very irregular outlines and appear rather crenated. In many instances, however, microglia resemble oligodendroglia and electron microscopists have as yet no reliable criteria to distinguish these two cell types.

1. Function. In case of injury or inflammatory reaction, the cells considered to be microglia round up and migrate to the injury site where they undergo cell division and become macrophages. The cells then become rod-like or distended as they become engorged with ingested debris.

D. Ependymal cells. These cells which line the ventricular surfaces may also be considered as supporting elements. There are regional modifications such that cells overlying white matter are low cuboidal to squamous while cells covering over grey matter may be columnar. At the rostral end of the cerebral aqueduct there is a rather specialized modification where the ependyma becomes pseudostratified and the cells are quite tall. The cells are filled with droplets which are apparently extruded or secreted into the cerebrospinal fluid. This is the subcommissural organ, which is just inferior to the posterior commissure. The ependymal cells lining the inferior aspect of the third ventricle adjacent to the periventricular cells of the hypothalamus are also believed to be modified to become secretory cells (tanycytes). The lateral surfaces of ependymal cells interdigitate with each other, but are not fused to prevent movement of solutes or particulate matter from the CSF into the brain parenchyma. Cilia are commonly found on the free surface of ependymal cells and have been shown to have a pattern of movement which would propel material from the lateral into the third ventricle and then down the cerebral aqueduct to the fourth ventricle and finally out into the subarachnoid spaces by exiting through the lateral foramen of Luschka. Microvilli are also present on the ventricular surface.

1. Functions.

a. Forms the germinal epithelium in fetal life.

b. Ciliary beating facilitates movement of materials out into the subarachnoid spaces.

c. Contributes to the formation of the cerebrospinal fluid as water moves from the brain parenchyma into the ventricular spaces.

d. May serve an active role in transporting certain wastes of brain metabolic activity from the zone of underlying glial processes.

Chapter 5

EXTERNAL SUPPORTING ELEMENTS

A. Phylogenetic development. While the meninges of lower animal forms appear grossly comparable to those of mammals, careful investigation reveals that they are not. In 1900—1901 Sterzi reported that the meninges of lower fishes such as cyclostomes and plagiostomes consisted of a single undifferentiated meninx, the meninx primitiva. He considered this to be the anlage of all three meningeal layers of mammals. Further, the vessels to the brain were observed to be limited to the meningeal envelope and did not penetrate into the brain (as in amphioxus).

1. Elasmobranchs (sharks). These still possess only a single membrane, but there are now many meningeal septa which penetrate the brain accompanied by vessels which are completely surrounded by the meninges and still do not directly contact the neural tissue.

2. Teleosts (bony fish). At this phylogenetic level the outer layer of the primitive meninx becomes thickened (Fig. 36), suggesting the development of the dura mater. Further, lateral thickenings in the meninx also appear, which are suggestive of the dentate ligaments of mammals. Vessels for the brain are within the meninx adjacent to the brain. There is also a well-developed extrameningeal venous plexus which may be the forerunner of the epidural venous plexus of mammals.

3. Amphibians. In the frog there is a complete separation between an outer thickened dural layer and an underlying leptomeningeal layer, the meninx secundaria. This appears to give rise to the pia and arachnoid layers in higher forms.

4. Reptiles. There is a further development of the intraparenchymal septa in reptiles which facilitates the entrance of the vessels. Leptomeningeal ligaments are more clearly evident. Major CNS vessels continue to be located in the meninges on the surface of the brain and the epidural plexus of veins continues to develop (Fig. 37).

5. Birds. As illustrated in the pigeon (Fig. 37), clefts begin to appear in the meninx secundaria foreshadowing the formation of a double-layered leptomeninges (pia and arachnoid). Vessels appear to be primarily in the deeper pial layer which is adherent to the brain.

6. Mammals. Three distinct meningeal layers are present upwards phylogenetically, starting with the marsupials, although the separation between pia and arachnoid never becomes complete. At numerous sites small strands, the arachnoid trabeculae, bind the two layers together. Furthermore, there may be numerous places where the separation into two layers is grossly incomplete.

7. In studying the development of the human meninges in the fetus, the various phases of the above phylogenetic series has been observed to be recapitulated. During advanced aging in man there is often some fusing of the leptomeninges which some workers feel may interfere with resorption of the cerebrospinal fluid.

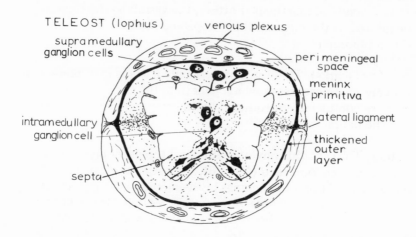

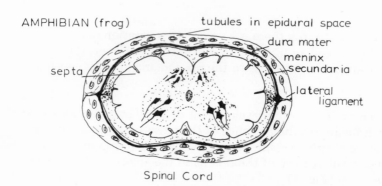

Fig. 36. The appearance of the meninges in teleosts as a single membrane with an external thickened layer and the meninges of amphibians as illustrated by the frog where an outer thickened dura mater has separated away from the underlying layer. Note the well-developed meningeal plexus of veins and a thickening in the meninx primitiva (lateral ligaments) foreshadowing the dentate ligaments.

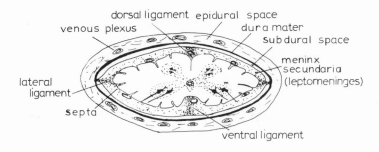

REPTILE (crocodile)

dorsal ligament epidural space
venous plexus dura mater
subdural space

meninx
secundaria
(leptomeninges)

lateral
ligament

septa

ventral ligament

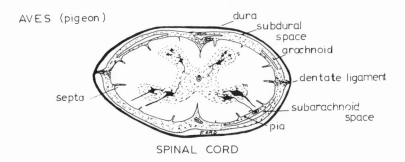

AVES (pigeon)

dura
subdural
space
arachnoid

dentate ligament

septa

subarachnoid
space

pia

SPINAL CORD

Fig. 37. The meninges of the reptile may be noted as having two distinct layers, a dura
mater and a meninx secundaria. Note the venous plexus in the epidural space and the
formation of lateral ligaments in the meninx secundaria. A separation of the meninx
secundaria into a pia mater and an outer arachnoid membrane becomes apparent in birds.

B. Dura mater.

1. Spinal cord. The dural envelope of the spinal cord (Figs 38 and 39)
invests the cord throughout its length, extending from the foramen magnum
caudally down over the cauda equina. The dura is adherent to the bodies of
the cervical vertebrae 2 and 3. At the level of the second sacral segment, the
dura becomes constricted into a thin filament which continues to descend and
finally fuses to the periosteum of the dorsal surface of the coccyx. This is the
filum of the dura mater. As the spinal nerves approach the dura they become
invested in a dural sheath which extends out laterally to fuse with the vertebral
periosteum at the intervertebral foramen. The spinal dura is surrounded by a
loose fibrous fatty tissue containing a well-developed plexus of veins, the
epidural venous plexus. The dura is attached ventrally by a series of irregular
poorly developed ligaments to the posterior longitudinal ligament of the
spinal column.

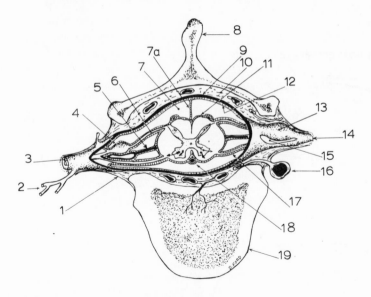

Fig. 38. A cross-sectional representation of the cervical spinal cord within the spinal canal surrounded by its meningeal sheaths. 1, region of dural fusion with periosteum; 2, lymphatic vessel draining perineuronal space; 3, perineuronal space; 4, subarachnoid space around dorsal root ganglion at point of fusion of pia and arachnoid; 5, dentate ligament; 6, dorsal root; 7, subarachnoid space; 7a, septum posticum; 8, spinal process; 9, dura mater; 10, epidural space; 11, pia mater; 12, arachnoid; 13, dorsal root ganglia sheathed with meninges; 14, spinal nerve; 15, interradicular foramen; 16, external vertebral vein; 17, ventral root; 18, anterior spinal artery; 19, vertebral body.

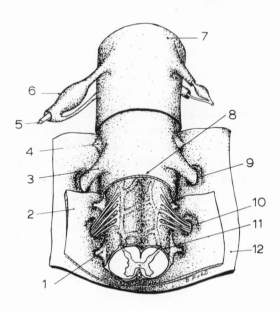

2. In the cranial cavity the dura becomes fused to the cranial periosteum. In so doing the epidural venous plexus appears to become compressed into a few large venous channels, the intradural venous sinuses. The inner layer of this double dural membrane becomes infolded to provide for a number of folds which project like septa between the major portions of the brain. These are the falx cerebri, falx cerebelli and tentorium cerebelli. Some of the major venous sinuses are located at the point where these folds turn away from the inner surface of the skull (see Figs 40—42).

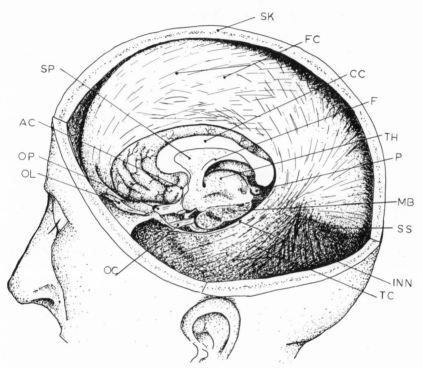

Fig. 40. A diagrammatic representation of the brain stem as it passes through the tentorial notch (incisura tentorii) in relation to the meninges to reach the diencephalon. AC, anterior commissure; CC, corpus callosum; F, fornix; FC, falx cerebri; INN, tentorial notch; MB, midbrain; OC, oculomotor nerve; P, pineal; SK, skull; SP, septum pellucidum; SS, region of straight sinus; TC, tentorium cerebelli; TH, thalamus; OL, olfactory bulb; OP, optic nerve.

Fig. 39. A representation of the spinal cord showing its relation to its three meningeal coverings. 1, dentate ligament passing through the arachnoid; 2, spinal arachnoid reflected; 3, dorsal root with accompanying sleeve of pia-arachnoid; 4, dentate ligament attaching to dura; 5, spinal nerve; 6, dorsal root ganglion with meningeal investment; 7, dura mater; 8, arachnoid; 9, dorsal root passing through the dura; 10, dorsal root passing through the arachnoid; 11, pia mater; 12, dura mater reflected.

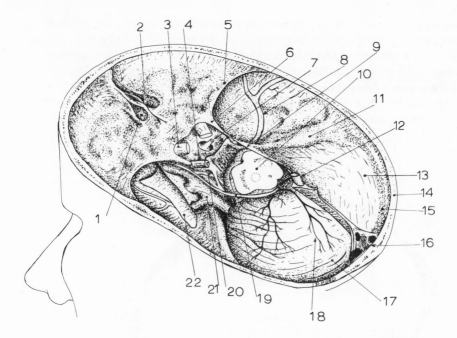

Fig. 41. The floor of the cranial cavity with the telencephalon and diencephalon removed. The left side of the tentorium cerebelli has also been reflected to expose the dorsum of the cerebellum. A flap of dura overlying the cavernous sinus has been reflected to demonstrate the three divisions of the trigeminal nerve and ganglia which lie in a dural cleft lateral to the sinus. 1, cavity in anterior cranial fossa for olfactory bulb; 2, crista galli; 3, optic nerve (II); 4, oculomotor nerve (III); 5, lesser wing of the sphenoid bone; 6, anterior clinoid process; 7, infundibulum projecting through diaphragma sellae; 8, middle meningeal artery; 9, tentorial notch (incisura); 10, midbrain; 11, petrous portion of temporal bone; 12, great cerebral vein (of Galen); 13, tentorium cerebelli; 14, occipital bone; 15, transverse sinus; 16, confluent sinus; 17, superior cerebellar surface; 18, superior cerebellar artery; 19, trochlear nerve (IV); 20, abducens nerve (VI); 21, trigeminal nerve (V); 22, dura reflected away from trigeminal nerve.

    a. The falx cerebri and falx cerebelli act as vertical struts projecting between the two halves of the brain in the midsagittal plane.

    b. The tentorium cerebelli lies in the horizontal plane, separating the cerebral and cerebellar hemispheres. It roofs over the posterior fossa of the skull, which contains the cerebellum, pons and medulla. The anterior margin of the tentorium is notched by the tentorial notch to permit the connection of the hind brain with the forebrain structures by the midbrain (mesencephalon).

C. Arachnoid. The arachnoid membrane is just deep to the dura mater and appears as a thin filmy layer of mesothelial cells separated from the pia by the

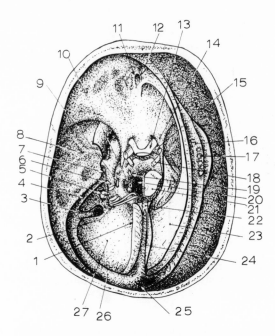

Fig. 42. A diagrammatic representation of a dissection of the interior of the skull. The telencephalon has been completely removed as has the left half of the brain stem. The major venous sinuses have been opened up on the left side. 1, cut edge of tentorium cerebelli; 2, glossopharyngeal, vagus and accessory nerves (IX, X, XI) exiting through the jugular foramen; 3, sigmoid sinus; 4, superior petrosal sinus; 5, facial and vestibulocochlear nerves (VII and VIII), exiting through internal auditory meatus; 6, trigeminal nerve (V); 7, cavernous sinus; 8, middle meningeal vessels in dura; 9, trochlear nerve (IV); 10, hypoglossal nerve (XII), exiting through hypoglossal foramen; 11, region of lamina cribrosa and olfactory bulb; 12, crista galli; 13, optic nerve (II) extending rostrally from chiasma; 14, anterior clinoid process; 15, internal carotid artery; 16, superior sagittal sinus; 17, arachnoid granulation; 18, oculomotor nerve (III); 19, abducens nerve (VI); 20, region of foramen magnum; 21, midbrain (mesencephalon); 22, great cerebral vein (of Galen); 23, falx cerebri; 24, straight sinus; 25, confluent sinus; 26, transverse sinus; 27, posterior cranial fossa.

subarachnoid space. This space is filled with cerebrospinal fluid. The entire space can be considered as being made up of cisterns, which often receive special names when they are of some size (Fig. 43).

1. Subarachnoid cistern. A general term referring to the entire subarachnoidal space.

2. The cistern of the great cerebral vein, cisterna ambiens, is a space extending rostrally from the level of the superior colliculus up over the roof of the third ventricle, being itself roofed over by the corpus callosum and the fornices.

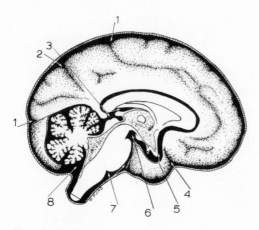

Fig. 43. A diagrammatic representation of the cisterns of the subarachnoid space. 1 and 2, subarachnoid cisterns as a general phenomenon not associated with a specific area of enlargement; 3, cistern of the great cerebral vein (cisterna ambiens); 4, cistern of the lateral fissure (rostral end); 5, chiasmatic cistern; 6, interpeduncular cistern; 7, pontine cistern; 8, cerebellomedullary cistern (cisterna magna).

3. The cisterna magna is that part of the subarachnoid between the dorsum of the medulla and the inferior aspect of the cerebellum.

4. The cisterna pontis extends along the ventral surface of the pons.

5. The interpeduncular cistern lies between the two crus cerebri of the midbrain.

6. The chiasmatic cistern is located in the region surrounding the optic chiasm.

7. The lateral cistern overlies the lateral fissure and extends down between the frontal and temporal lobes to the insula.

D. Arachnoid granulations. These are rather nodular outpocketings of arachnoid tissue which project primarily into the superior sagittal sinus and provide for one of the avenues whereby cerebrospinal fluid is drained out into the venous system. There are, in addition, pia-arachnoid cuffs which form around exiting nerve fibers as they pass through the intervertebral foramina or the foramina of the skull. Cerebrospinal fluid has been observed to pass through these cuffs into the perineuronal spaces, which are in turn drained by lymphatic vessels.

E. Pia mater. This leptomeningeal layer is closely adherent to the surface of the brain and extends into every space, sulcus or fissure. Since the arachnoid membrane bridges over these spaces, the subarachnoid space becomes enlarged at these points to form cisterns. The mesothelial elements of the pia resemble those of the arachnoid. Lateral projections occur as the dentate ligaments which attach to the dura. A dorsal projection (septum posticum) attaches the pia to the arachnoid membrane.

F. The relations of the leptomeninges to the blood vessels. As observed in many mammalian forms, the blood vessels traverse the arachnoid spaces supported by trabeculae, which blend with the adventitia of the vessels. An attenuated layer of leptomeningeal cytoplasm covers over the vessels. As the vessels penetrate the brain, they are accompanied by a surface layer of lepto-meningeal cells for a short distance and by a very short projection of the subarachnoid space around the larger vessels. The layer of pia covering the brain surface also projects down into this space and very soon fuses to the layer of meningeal cells covering the vessel. The subpial layer of astrocyte foot processes also follows the vessel into the brain forming a cuff around the pial layer. The meningeal layer ends at the level of the capillary, but the glial cuff around the vessel continues, covering up to 85% of the surface of the capillary. At this point there is nothing comparable to the perivascular space described by earlier investigators. Such a space is limited to the very short segment of the vessel just as it perforates into the brain parenchyma.

Chapter 6

CORTEX

Cerebral cortex. There are two basic types of cortex in the cerebrum: isocortex (neo- and paleocortex) having six layers and allocortex (archicortex) having three layers. The allocortex consists of the hippocampus and dentate gyrus and an adjacent area limited to the cortex of the uncus and rostral hippocampal gyrus. The latter two areas are not strictly three-layered, but intermediate in that there are fewer cell types than seen in the six-layered cortex elsewhere. The rest of the cortex of the cerebrum is of the six-layered variety (see Fig. 44). Phylogenetically, archicortex is the oldest and neocortex

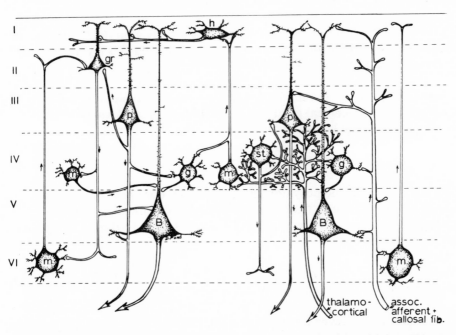

Fig. 44. A diagrammatic representation (after Lorente de Nó, 1949) of the cell layers and interconnections of the neocerebral cortex. The layers are numbered I through VI. I, molecular layer; II, outer granule cell layer; III, outer pyramidal cell layer; IV, inner granule cell layer; V, inner pyramidal cell layer; VI, polymorphic cell layer. B, giant pyramidal cell (Betz cell); g, Golgi-type cell; gr, granule cell; h, horizontal cell; m, cell of Martinotti; p, pyramidal cell; st, stellate cell. Thalamocortical refers to projections from the diencephalon to the cortex; assoc. afferent + callosal fib. refers to short and long associational fibers and commissural fibers which terminate in the cortex.

the most recently acquired. In man the allocortex is represented by the hippocampus and dentate gyrus. The paleocortex is restricted to a small area adjacent to the hippocampal structure in the piriform area. The remainder and by far the greater part of the cortex of man is neocortex.

A. Layers of the isocortex.

1. Layer I. The molecular layer which contains few neurons (horizontal cells and small granule cells) plus dendritic and axonal processes from the deeper layers.

2. Layer II. The external granule layer is made up of small pyramidal-shaped neurons and granule cells, whose axons end in layers IV, V and VI.

3. Layer III. The external pyramidal layer is made up of small pyramidal cells which get progressively larger the deeper the progression into the cortex. Their axons leave the cortex to project to adjacent cortical areas.

4. Layer IV. The inner granule layer contains mostly granule, Golgi or stellate cells and a few small pyramidal cells. Axons from this layer primarily return to more superficial layers or to layers V and VI.

5. Layer V. The inner pyramidal cell layer contains large pyramidal cells, particularly in the precentral gyrus (primary motor cortex), where some of them are exceptionally large and are known as the giant pyramidal cells (Betz cells). These are the primary projection neurons whose axons leave the cortex as long association, commissural or projection fibers.

6. Layer VI. This is the polymorphic layer which contains cells of many sizes and shapes (spindle or fusiform cells, cells of Martinotti, etc.). Note that many cells of this layer have axons which pass back to the surface of the cortex.

B. The six-layered cortex may be subdivided into layers which are primarily afferent or receptor layers and into efferent or projection layers.

1. Afferent layers. Layer IV contains a large ramification of axonal terminals arising from the dorsal thalamus and metathalamus. This establishes layer IV as the primary receptive layer of the cortex. The postcentral gyrus, superior transverse temporal gyrus and the cortex surrounding the calcarine fissure are particularly well-developed in this layer.

2. Efferent layers. Layer II contains cells which project to other layers within the adjacent cortex, but do not project out into the subjacent white

matter. Layers III, V and VI contain cells which project to other cortical areas or to subcortical areas. Layer V is the primary layer for subcortical projection, giving rise to fibers entering the internal capsule for distribution to the thalamus, brain stem and spinal cord.

C. Layers of the allocortex (hippocampus and dentate gyrus).

1. Molecular layer. This is comparable to that of isocortex in having few cells and many fibers coming in from other areas.

2. The pyramidal layer contains both large and small pyramidal cells in a densely packed layer of cells. These are often called double pyramidal cells because of the extensive dendritic ramifications which arise from both ends of the cell.

3. The axons of these cells enter into the fornix via the alveus and project to the mammillary bodies, preoptic areas, thalamus and midbrain.

4. The polymorphic layer, as before, contains a number of different cell types including modified pyramidal cells. It is not nearly as densely populated a layer as the pyramidal layer.

5. In the dentate gyrus a layer of granule cells is substituted for the pyramidal cells which occur in the hippocampus. The axons of these cells then project through the polymorphic layer of the dentate gyrus to reach the hippocampus where they terminate on the dendrites of hippocampal pyramidal cells.

D. Regional differences. Various investigators (Brodmann, Vogt, Von Economo, Bailey) studied the cerebral cortex and concluded it could be mapped into different regions based on variations in the types of cells present, their number and size (architectonics). After mapping, a variety of numbering schemes were devised to indicate each area (Figs 45 and 46). As originally described, these numbered areas were believed to differ discretely from each other. However, as indicated in the figures, it is more likely that if such anatomical maps can be drawn, the individual areas will blend or overlap. Clark has called attention to the inexactness of how these measurements were originally made with the result that the numbering systems are useful today primarily as a shorthand for referring to various specific regions. Perhaps, of all the classifications, that of Von Economo who described only five general types of cortex (based on cell populations) is most useful. These are the agranular, frontal, parietal, polar and granular cortices.

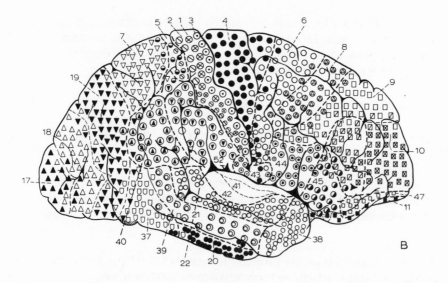

Fig. 45. A schematic modification of the Brodmann numbering scheme for cellular architectural differences from one area of the lateral surface of the cortex to another. Note that the symbols overlap each other to indicate that these regional boundaries are not sharply delimited.

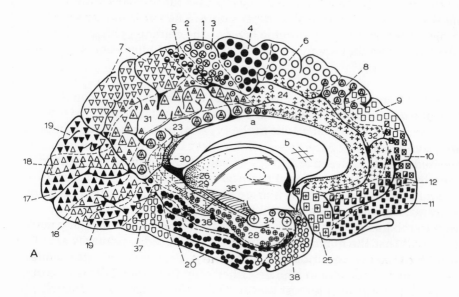

Fig. 46. A schematic modification of the Brodmann numbering scheme for the architectural distribution of various cortical neurons underlying the midsagittal surface of the cerebrum. C.C., corpus callosum; S.P., septum pellucidum.

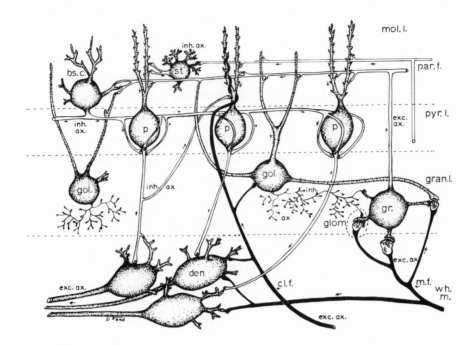

Fig. 47. A diagrammatic representation (based on Eccles *et al.*, 1967) of the cell types and interconnections which occur in the cerebellar cortex, including Purkinje cell projections to the cells of the deep cerebellar nuclei. bs.c., basket cell; cl.f., climbing fiber; den, cell of the dentate nucleus; exc. ax., excitatory axon; glom., glomerulus; gol., Golgi-type cell; gr., granule cell; gran.l., granule cell layer; inh. ax., inhibitory axon; m.f., mossy fiber; mol.l., molecular layer; p, Purkinje cell; par.f., parallel fiber; pyr. l., Purkinje cell layer; st, stellate cell; wh. m., white matter.

E. Cerebellar cortex. The cerebellar cortex contains only three layers: molecular, Purkinje and granular (Fig. 47).

1. The molecular layer contains the dendritic processes of Purkinje cells, the axons of the granule cells (parallel fibers), stellate cells and basket cells. It is in this layer that the climbing fibers which arise from the inferior olive terminate by wrapping around the Purkinje cell dendrites. They have also been observed to have terminals on every other cell type of the cerebellar cortex. Parallel fibers arising from granule cells run parallel to the surface of the cerebellar folia and are strung out across the Purkinje dendritic trees like wires.

2. The Purkinje cell layer is only one cell layer thick and contains the flask-shaped Purkinje cells whose axons provide the only efferent output from the cerebellar cortex. Synapses of basket cells are made at the base of the Purkinje

cell in this layer and have an inhibitory effect on the propagation of impulses from the Purkinje cell.

3. The granule cell layer contains granule and Golgi II cells. Mossy fibers arising from the cells of the spinal cord, pons and medulla which project to the cerebellum terminate in this layer. Dendrites of the Golgi II cells can be observed being contacted by the parallel fibers, climbing fibers and by mossy fibers. Their axons, in turn, act at the level of synapse of the mossy fiber (axon) with the dendrite of the granule cell to provide for postsynaptic inhibition.

4. The cells of one of the deep cerebellar nuclei (dentate nucleus) are illustrated in Fig. 47 to indicate that they are the final efferent elements of the cerebellum, relaying the inhibitory influence of the cerebellar cortex to other CNS levels. Note that these cells also receive an input from the climbing and mossy fibers. It is interesting to note that, if the cerebellar cortex is removed neurosurgically, the resulting ataxia (dyssynergia) is less if the deep nuclei are not damaged.

Chapter 7

WHITE MATTER

A. Cerebrum. The cerebral white matter is made up of short and long association fibers connecting various gyri or lobes to each other, and commissural fibers which connect comparable areas of the two hemispheres (anterior, hippocampal and corpus callosum), or the two sides of the brain stem (posterior, hypothalamic, habenular). The anterior commissure of the spinal cord is somewhat different in that it consists of fibers arising from cells of the dorsal horn which project rostrally to different areas of the CNS. There are also in this commissure fibers arising from the medial ventral horn cells which terminate within the same or neighboring spinal segments. Finally, there are some commissural elements derived from the anterior corticospinal tract. A significant component of the white matter is the projection fiber system which interconnects the diencephalon and basal ganglia with the cortex or which arises from the cortex and projects to the brain stem or spinal cord.

B. Cerebellum. A great part of the cerebellar white matter comes from its three pairs of peduncles (the inferior and middle which are afferent to the hemisphere and the superior which is efferent from the dentate, globose and emboliform nuclei). Another large contribution is provided by the axons of the Purkinje cells as they project into the white matter to terminate on the deep nuclei. Finally, there is a relatively small group of fibers associated with the fastigial nuclei connecting them to the vestibular nuclei. These are the juxtarestiform body and the uncinate fasciculus which collectively form the fastigiobulbar tract.

C. Brain stem. The bundles of white matter seen either grossly or on Pal-Weigert stained slides consist essentially of the long projecting ascending and descending systems which either project through cellular areas or are appended onto the outer surface (pes pedunculi).

D. Spinal cord. The white matter of the cord is all peripherally located and consists of short association fibers (fasciculus proprius) which connect adjacent levels of the cord, longer association bundles which project up or down the various funiculi to interconnect further segments of the cord, or very long projection systems which project to supracord levels or which enter the cord from higher levels. The entering and exiting nerve roots will also contribute to the white matter of the cord.

Chapter 8

VASCULAR SYSTEM

A careful study of the vascular system of the CNS reveals that it is essentially segmentally organized. If the CNS is extended (Fig. 48) so that all the components are in their relative embryologic position end to end, the cerebral hemisphere is seen to be rostral to the basal ganglia, which are in turn rostral to the thalamus, etc. The subsequent distribution of the arteries is then such that the forebrain (telencephalon-diencephalon) is supplied by the four major branches of the internal carotid artery in such a fashion that the more anterior parts are supplied by the anterior cerebral artery and the most posterior parts by the posterior cerebral artery. Note in the figure that the posterior cerebral artery is shown arising from the internal carotid artery. This complies with the embryologic origin of the vessel which only secondarily during development comes to receive its major arterial blood contribution from the vertebral-basilar complex. Indeed, in many adult brains this primitive condition is partially maintained. In a very few rare cases (less than 0.5%) a Circle of Willis is not even partially formed. In these instances the diencephalon is supplied by vessels arising from the internal carotid arteries or from the posterior cerebral arteries which in turn also derive their blood completely from the internal carotid arteries and supply the posterior aspect of the cerebral hemisphere. The hindbrain structures (medulla, pons-cerebellum) and midbrain are then supplied by the four major branches of the vertebral-basilar arterial complex (not illustrated in the figure) in a continued segmental sequence. The spinal arteries then logically follow segmentally.

In analyzing the relative position of the arteries to the veins on the surface of the brain, it may be observed that the arteries approach the brain from its ventral aspect and that the veins tend to drain dorsally. This is particularly true of the veins draining the deep nuclear structures (diencephalon and basal ganglia) wherein the venous effluent eventually passes into the great cerebral vein (of Galen) on the dorsal aspect of the neural tube. Of course, all the venous blood must finally reach a ventral position relative to the brain in order to leave the cranial cavity.

A. Arterial development. Initially, the brain receives two distinct separate arterial supplies (Fig. 49). There is the internal carotid artery which terminates on the surface of the brain as the primitive maxillary, primitive olfactory and posterior cerebral (caudal branch) arteries. Another pair of vessels ascends in close apposition to the ventral brain surface to terminate in the region of the midbrain. These are the longitudinal neural arteries. Each of these arteries

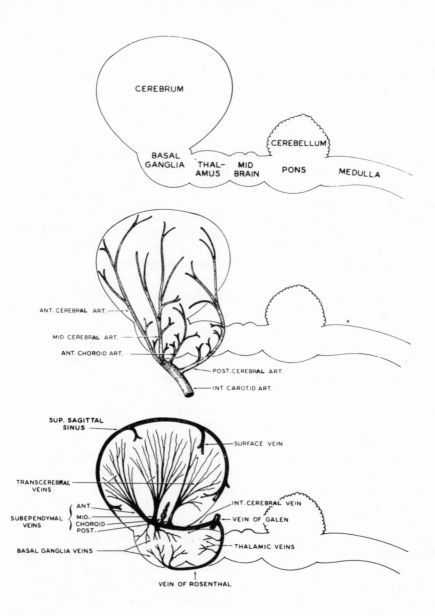

Fig. 48. The figure at the top illustrates the major components of the CNS as a series of segmentally related structures. The illustration in the middle demonstrates the projection of the four major arterial trunks derived from the embryologic internal carotid artery into those parts of the CNS formed from the prosencephalon (cerebral hemisphere, basal ganglia and diencephalon). The bottom figure illustrates the venous drainage from the same prosencephalic structures. Note that the anterior subependymal vein is often referred to as the septal vein and that the middle and posterior subependymal veins are usually linked together to form the thalamostriate vein (vena terminalis). (Unpublished figure generously provided by H. Kaplan.)

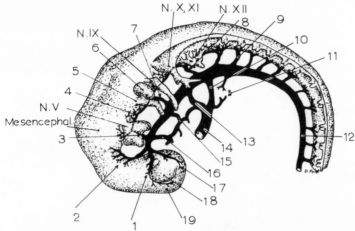

Fig. 49. A diagrammatic representation of the very primitive arterial supply of the CNS of the 4.0 mm embryo. 1, cranial division of the internal carotid artery (primitive olfactory artery); 2, diencephalon with the caudally directed branch of the primitive internal carotid artery (the primitive posterior cerebral artery); 3, primitive trigeminal artery; 4, longitudinal neural artery; 5, facial and vestibulocochlear nerves; 6, otic vesicle; 7, primitive otic artery; 8, primitive hypoglossal artery; 9, first cervical segmental artery; 10, fourth aortic arch; 11, pulmonary arch in formation; 12, paired aortae; 13, third aortic arch; 14, arterial trunk; 15, hyoid artery (second aortic arch); 16, mandibular artery (first aortic arch); 17, primitive maxillary artery; 18, optic vesicle; 19, telencephalon.

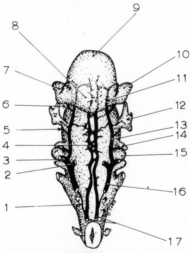

Fig. 50. A frontal view of the arterial supply to the CNS of a 6.0 mm embryo. 1, dwindling primitive hypoglossal artery; 2, fourth aortic arch; 3, third aortic arch; 4, developing basilar artery; 5, remnant of the mandibular artery; 6, primitive maxillary artery; 7, primitive olfactory artery (cranial portion of internal carotid artery); 8, prosencephalon; 9, mesencephalon; 10, optic vesicle; 11, developing proximal stem of the posterior cerebral artery from the caudal division of the internal carotid artery; 12, dwindling primitive trigeminal artery; 13, internal carotid artery; 14, hyoid artery; 15, otic vesicle; 16, paired aortae; 17, bilateral longitudinal neural artery.

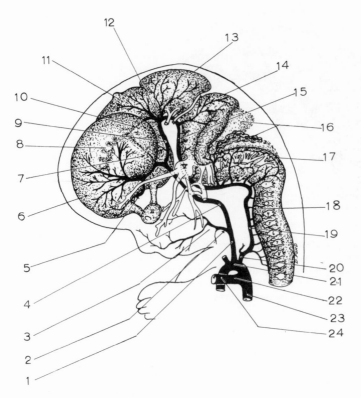

Fig. 51. The lateral aspect of the arteries to the CNS in the 24 mm embryo. 1, common carotid artery; 2, external carotid artery; 3, external maxillary artery; 4, internal carotid artery; 5, anterior cerebral artery; 6, telencephalon with branches of the middle cerebral artery; 7, anterior choroid artery; 8, choroid plexus of lateral ventricle; 9, proximal stem of posterior cerebral artery (posterior communicating artery); 10, posterior choroid artery; 11, diencephalic arteries; 12, mesencephalic artery; 13, tectal branches of the mesencephalic artery; 14, superior cerebellar artery; 15, basilar artery; 16, choroid plexus in roof of fourth ventricle; 17, arterial plexus giving rise to the posterior inferior cerebellar artery; 18, anterior spinal artery; 19, vertebral artery; 20, subclavian artery; 21, aortic arch; 22, ductus arteriosus; 23, aorta; 24, pulmonary artery.

will provide for the three cerebellar arteries and then most rostrally for a mesencephalic artery. The two arterial systems are joined together, as they run parallel to each other along the neural tube, by primitive vessels which usually regress. These are the primitive hypoglossal, otic and trigeminal arteries. When viewed from the ventral aspect (Fig. 50), the two longitudinal neural arteries can be seen to be approaching each other and establishing a number of interconnecting rami. The two vessels will fuse at this level to form the basilar artery (arteria basilaris). The remaining caudal segments of the longitudinal neural arteries remain in the adult as the vertebral arteries.

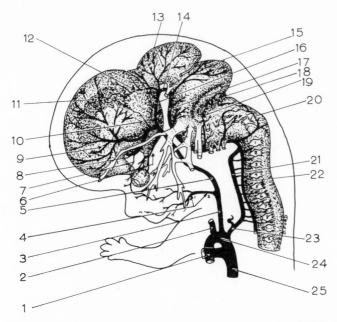

Fig. 52. The lateral aspect of the arterial supply to the CNS in the 40 mm embryo.
1, pulmonary artery; 2, innominate artery; 3, common carotid artery; 4, external maxillary artery (1) arising from the external carotid artery; 5, internal carotid artery; 6, ophthalmic artery; 7, primitive olfactory artery; 8, anterior cerebral artery; 9, middle cerebral artery; 10, anterior choroid artery; 11, choroid plexus in lateral ventricle; 12, posterior choroid artery; 13, tectal branches of the mesencephalic artery; 14, mesencephalic artery; 15, superior cerebellar artery; 16, proximal stem of the posterior cerebral artery (posterior communicating artery); 17, basilar artery; 18, choroid plexus of fourth ventricle; 19, stem of anterior inferior cerebellar artery; 20, stem of posterior inferior cerebellar artery; 21, vertebral artery; 22, anterior spinal artery; 23, subclavian artery; 24, aortic arch; 25, aorta.

As development proceeds, the mesencephalic artery fuses with the posterior cerebral artery (Figs 51—53) to form a vascular circle at the base of the brain (Circle of Willis). Usually the mesencephalic arterial stem comes to be the most important in providing blood to be distributed through the posterior cerebral artery. By custom we have come to call the vessel which links the mesencephalic and internal carotid arteries the posterior communicating artery (arteria communicans posterior), whereas it may more properly be termed the proximal stem of the posterior cerebral artery. Elements of the original embryologic mesencephalic artery may still be discerned supplying the midbrain. Note that as development proceeds the arterial stems grow out over the surface of the brain. Arterial collateral links are finally established between the major surface vessels and through the Circle of Willis. The perforating vessels which arise from the surface network plexus of vessels are functionally end arteries. That is, there are no effective functional collateral connections between adjacent cell groups within the brain. Finally, the major surface vessels appear as illustrated in Fig. 54. By this time each major vessel may be defined as having three basic components.

1. A short proximal stem which gives off perforators to medially placed deep nuclear structures.

2. A more lateral or distal stem which gives off perforators to the more laterally placed deep nuclear structures.

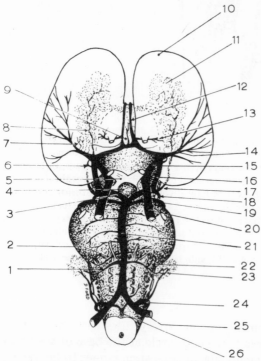

Fig. 53. The anterior aspect of the CNS of the 40 mm embryo, demonstrating the formation of the Circle of Willis. 1, stem of anterior inferior cerebellar artery; 2, labyrinthine artery; 3, mesencephalic artery; 4, pituitary; 5, optic chiasm; 6, anterior choroid artery; 7, lenticulostriate perforators (proximal and distal perforators) of the middle cerebral artery; 8, choroid plexus lateral ventricle; 9, artery of the corpus callosum arising from the anterior communicating artery; 13, medial striate artery (Heubner-distal perforator); 14, middle cerebral artery; 15, internal carotid artery; 16, proximal stem of posterior cerebral artery (posterior communicating artery); 17, posterior choroid artery; 18, posterior cerebral artery; 19, superior cerebellar artery; 20, internal carotid artery; 21, basilar artery; 22, labyrinthine artery arising from the anterior inferior cerebellar artery; 23, choroid plexus of fourth ventricle; 24, stem of posterior inferior cerebellar and posterior spinal arteries; 25, vertebral artery; 26, anterior spinal artery.

90

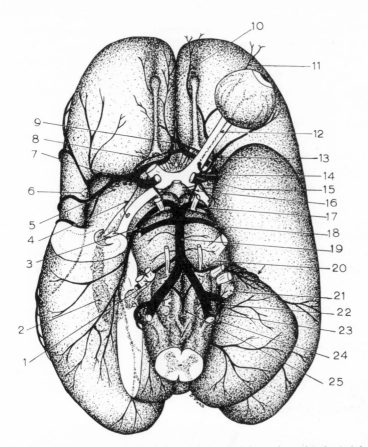

Fig. 54. The distribution of the major arterial trunks at birth. 1, labyrinthine artery arising from the anterior inferior cerebellar artery; 2, choroid plexus of lateral ventricle; 3, posterior cerebral artery; 4, anterior choroid artery; 5, proximal and distal perforators (lenticulostriate) of the middle cerebral artery; 6, candelabra (insular) branches of the middle cerebral artery; 7, middle cerebral artery; 8, medial striate artery (Heubner-distal perforator); 9, anterior cerebral artery; 10, supratrochlear artery; 11, supraorbital artery; 12, central retinal artery; 13, lacrimal artery; 14, stem of ophthalmic artery; 15, internal carotid artery; 16, proximal stem of posterior cerebral artery (posterior communicating artery); 17, posterior cerebral artery; 18, superior cerebellar artery; 19, basilar artery; 20, anterior inferior cerebellar artery; 21, choroid plexus of fourth ventricle; 22, posterior inferior cerebellar artery; 23, vertebral artery; 24, posterior spinal artery; 25, anterior spinal artery.

3. A cortical arborization or network which provides for cortical perforators.

B. Development of the venous system. The venous system develops in a series of stages comparable to those of the arteries. However, the adult configuration is attained somewhat later. In the 2—3 mm embryo there is a very simple drainage pattern consisting of a primordial hindbrain channel lying directly

on the dorsal aspect of the neural tube. This is continuous with the anterior
cardinal veins. This primordial channel plays no role in the final circulation
of the brain, but is made up of the proliferative endothelium from which pial
arteries and veins are derived. By the 5 mm stage this tube has disappeared,
to be replaced by a more lateral channel, the primary head sinus, from which
arise various dural plexuses which project to the surface of the brain (Fig. 55).
As the brain continues to develop, a considerable plexus of veins forms over
the surface of the brain which drain into sinuses which come to be positioned
between the true dura and the periosteal dura (Figs 56—58). At birth, the
complex of large intradural sinuses and veins is essentially complete (Figs
59—62). At this point veins draining the surface of the brain, as well as the
veins draining deep nuclei, empty into the intradural sinuses (superior and
inferior sagittal sinuses, straight sinus, confluent sinus, transverse sinus,
superior and inferior petrosal sinuses, and the cavernous sinus). Note that
various portions of some of these sinuses have been observed to be atretic at
autopsy (Kaplan and Browder). For example, the rostral third of the superior

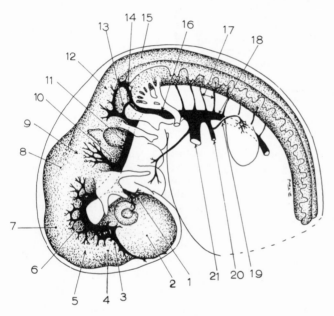

Fig. 55. A lateral view of the distribution of the early primitive veins draining the CNS of
the 5 mm embryo. 1, primitive maxillary vein; 2, telencephalon; 3, developing primitive
marginal sinus; 4, diencephalon; 5, anterior dural plexus; 6, stem of anterior dural plexus;
7, mesencephalon; 8, metencephalon; 9, middle dural plexus; 10, stem of middle dural
plexus; 11, primary head sinus; 12, posterior dural plexus; 13, secondary anastomosis;
14, stem of posterior dural plexus; 15, myelencephalon; 16, anterior cardinal vein;
17, intersegmental veins; 18, posterior cardinal vein; 19, primitive vein for arm bud;
20, thoraco-epigastric vein; 21, common cardinal vein.

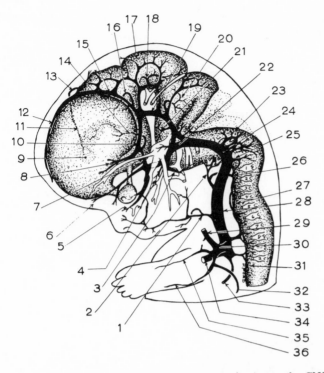

Fig. 56. A lateral view of the distribution of veins to the CNS and head of the 24 mm embryo. 1, common facial vein; 2, ventral myelencephalic vein; 3, remnant of primitive head sinus; 4, pharyngeal vein; 5, maxillary vein; 6, primitive supraorbital vein; 7, dwindling stem of anterior dural plexus; 8, superficial middle cerebral vein; 9, choroid plexus; 10, tentorial sinus; 11, internal cerebral vein; 12, superior sagittal sinus; 13, primitive straight sinus; 14, ventral diencephalic vein; 15, marginal sinus; 16, dorsal diencephalic vein; 17, tentorial plexus; 18, mesencephalic vein; 19, primitive transverse sinus; 20, dorsal metencephalic vein; 21, ventral metencephalic vein; 22, pro-otic sinus (stem of middle dural plexus); 23, posterior dural plexus; 24, sigmoid sinus; 25, primitive emissary vein (condylaris); 26, primitive hypoglossal emissary vein; 27, vertebral vein; 28, internal jugular vein; 29, external jugular vein; 30, subclavian vein; 31, superior intercostal vein; 32, thoraco-epigastric vein; 33, coronary sinus; 34, left innominate vein; 35, cephalic vein; 36, ulnar vein.

sagittal sinus may be so restricted in size as to be nonfunctional, in which case the frontal polar veins run caudally over the dorsum of the hemisphere to empty into the sinus where it becomes patent. These areas of atresia do not seem to have compromised cerebral blood flow to a sufficient extent to have produced neurologic symptoms since alternative routes of venous drainage appear to have been successfully utilized.

1. Cerebellar veins also drain into the intradural sinuses at six relatively specific areas. Anterior cerebellar veins drain into the two superior petrosal

sinuses and into the great cerebral vein or straight sinus. Veins along the posterior margin of the cerebellum drain into the transverse sinuses and confluent sinus.

2. Veins draining the ventral aspect of the brain stem frequently coalesce into a large vein which drains into the superior petrosal sinus, though there may be many small veins accomplishing this purpose. These ventral brain stem veins also frequently unite with the basal vein and thus may finally drain dorsally into the great cerebral vein.

3. The deep veins draining the dorsal aspect of the diencephalon and basal ganglia may be visualized if the cerebral hemispheres are pulled apart and the

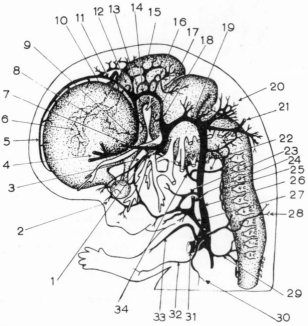

Fig. 57. A lateral view of the venous drainage from the CNS and head of the 40 mm embryo. 1, cavernous sinus; 2, supratrochlear-facial vein anastomosis; 3, stem of superior ophthalmic vein; 4, middle cerebral vein; 5, superior sagittal sinus; 6, choroid veins; 7, middle meningeal sinus; 8, internal cerebral vein; 9, ventral diencephalic vein; 10, straight sinus; 11, primitive marginal sinus; 12, dorsal diencephalic vein; 13, mesencephalic vein; 14, primitive transverse sinus; 15, tentorial plexus; 16, dorsal metencephalic vein; 17, ventral metencephalic vein; 18, pro-otic sinus; 19, sigmoid sinus; 20, posterior dural plexus; 21, occipital vein; 22, primitive hypoglossal and condylar emissary veins; 23, common facial vein; 24, external jugular vein; 25, vertebral vein; 26, internal jugular vein; 27, subclavian vein; 28, deep cervical vein; 29, superior intercostal vein; 30, thoraco-epigastric vein; 31, innominate vein; 32, ulnar vein; 33, cephalic vein; 34, ventral myelencephalic vein.

94

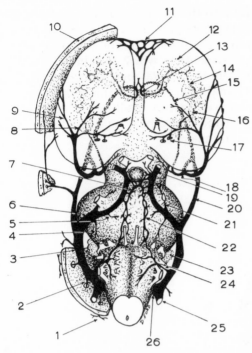

Fig. 58. An anterior view of the veins draining the CNS of the 40 mm embryo. 1, condylar emissary vein; 2, mastoid emissary vein; 3, sigmoid sinus; 4, remnant of head sinus; 5, pharyngeal vein; 6, pro-otic sinus; 7, cavernous sinus; 8, deep middle cerebral vein; 9, superficial middle cerebral vein; 10, frontal bone; 11, developing superior sagittal sinus; 12, choroid plexus of lateral ventricle; 13, internal cerebral vein; 14, posterior choroid vein; 15, marginal sinus; 16, anterior choroid vein; 17, inferior striate veins; 18, ventral diencephalic vein; 19, stem of the superior ophthalmic vein; 20, transverse sinus; 21, ventral metencephalic vein; 22, inferior petrosal sinus; 23, choroid plexus of fourth ventricle; 24, ventral myelencephalic vein; 25, internal jugular vein; 26, stem of posterior dural plexus.

corpus callosum removed (Fig. 61). In so doing, the two internal cerebral veins which empty into the great cerebral vein will be exposed lying along the roof of the third ventricle in the cistern of the great cerebral vein. Three major groups of veins join in the roof of the foramen of Monro to form the internal cerebral veins. These are the

    a. Septal veins.
    b. Choroidal veins.
    c. Thalamostriate (terminal) veins (or subependymal vein).

4. Veins draining the ventral aspect of the basal ganglia may be observed draining into the deep middle cerebral vein as it passes along the surface of the anterior perforated substance just deep to the middle cerebral artery. The

rostral aspects of the basal ganglia drain into the anterior cerebral vein which is just deep to the anterior cerebral artery. (The preoptic and rostral hypothalamic structures would also drain into the anterior cerebral vein.) These two veins join to form the basal vein (of Rosenthal) which runs back along the optic tract receiving contributions from the ventral diencephalon (hypothalamus). It passes dorsally around the midbrain to empty finally into the great cerebral vein (of Galen). In its course around the midbrain, it receives mesencephalic, cerebellar and occipital venous contributions, as well as further diencephalic rami from the caudal thalamus.

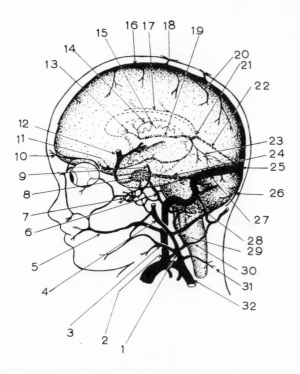

Fig. 59. A lateral view of the veins draining the head and CNS at birth. 1, external jugular vein; 2, internal jugular vein; 3, anterior jugular vein; 4, superficial temporal vein; 5, anterior facial vein; 6, inferior petrosal sinus; 7, pterygoid plexus; 8, cavernous sinus; 9, middle meningeal vein; 10, supraorbital vein; 11, anterior cerebral vein; 12, superficial middle cerebral vein; 13, vein of the septum pellucidum (anterior subependymal vein); 14, thalamostriate vein (middle and posterior subependymal veins together, sometimes called vena terminalis); 15, superior choroid veins; 16, superior sagittal sinus; 17, inferior sagittal sinus; 18, emissary vein; 19, internal cerebral vein; 20, superior cerebral vein; 21, great cerebral vein (of Galen); 22, straight sinus; 23, superior cerebellar veins; 24, superior petrosal sinus; 25, confluent sinus; 26, occipital sinus; 27, transverse sinus; 28, sigmoid sinus; 29, vertebral vein; 30, deep cervical vein; 31, transverse scapular vein; 32, subscapular vein.

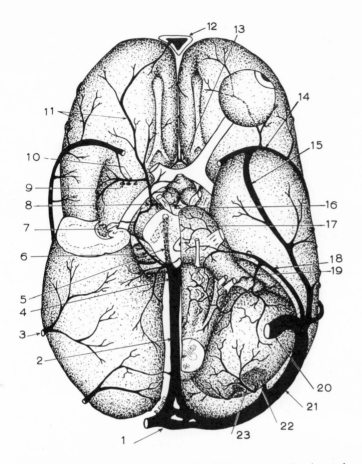

Fig. 60. The ventral aspect of brain of the newborn (gyri not shown) illustrating the distribution of the major drainage veins. 1, confluent sinus; 2, straight sinus; 3, an inferior cerebral vein; 4, great cerebral vein (of Galen); 5, internal cerebral vein; 6, basal vein (of Rosenthal); 7, choroid plexus of lateral ventricle and anterior choroid vein; 8, basal vein; 9, inferior striate veins; 10, deep middle cerebral vein; 11, orbital veins; 12, superior sagittal sinus; 13, anterior cerebral vein with an anterior communicating vein; 14, superficial middle cerebral vein; 15, remnant of tentorial sinus; 16, interpeduncular veins; 17, ventral metencephalic (pontine) vein; 18, superior petrosal sinus; 19, anterior cerebellar vein; 20, internal jugular vein; 21, transverse sinus; 22, cerebellar tentorial sinus; 23, posterior cerebellar vein.

Note that the two anterior cerebral veins are joined by what could be called an anterior communicating vein and that various elements of the basal veins anastomose with each other on the surface of the diencephalon or in the interpeduncular fossa. This serves to form a venous circle in some ways comparable to the Circle of Willis.

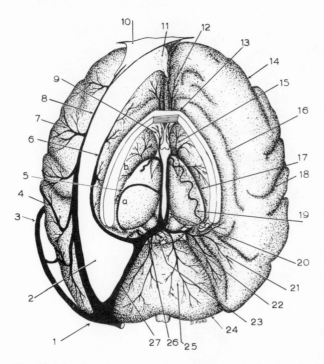

Fig. 61. The dorsal aspect of the brain with the hemispheres pulled apart and corpus callosum removed to expose the deep veins of the brain. 1, confluent sinus; 2, falx cerebri; 3, transverse sinus; 4, superior cerebral vein; 5, posterior subependymal vein (posterior part of thalamostriate vein); 6, inferior sagittal sinus; 7, superior cerebral vein; 8, superior sagittal sinus; 9, septal vein (anterior subependymal vein); 10, dura mater; 11, crista galli; 12, anterior cerebral vein; 13, corpus callosum; 14, cerebral hemisphere; 15, subependymal veins draining caudate nucleus; 16, sulcus cinguli; 17, middle subependymal vein (thalamo-striate vein or vena terminalis); 18, central sulcus; 19, choroid vein; 20, internal cerebral vein; 21, occipital veins draining into basal vein; 22, basal vein; 23, mesencephalic veins draining into the great cerebral vein; 24, cerebellum; 25, superior cerebellar veins; 26, great cerebral vein (of Galen); 27, straight sinus; a, thalamus; b, nucleus caudatus.

5. Transcerebral veins. These are small vessels about 15 to 20 microns in diameter which radiate out from the subependymal veins in the wall of the lateral ventricles. They connect with the cerebral cortical venous drainage. Thus, the cortical capillaries may drain either into the surface cortical veins or via the transcerebral veins which in turn drain into the internal cerebral veins.

C. Figs 63—66 summarize the distribution of arteries to the forebrain components of the brain and represent the distributions of the four vessels which originally arise from the terminal end of the internal carotid artery. The distribution of the arteries to the midbrain is illustrated in Fig. 66 as arising from what may be called the mesencephalic component of the posterior

98

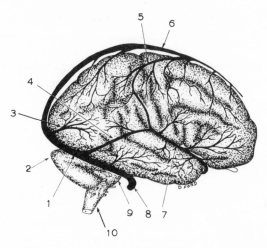

Fig. 62. A lateral view of the venous drainage of the CNS showing the major anastomotic connections. 1, transverse sinus; 2, cerebellum; 3, inferior cerebral veins; 4, inferior anastomotic vein (of Labbé); 5, superior anastomotic vein (of Trollard); 6, superior sagittal sinus; 7, superficial middle cerebral vein which also drains medially into the cavernous sinus; 8, sigmoid sinus; 9, pons; 10, medulla.

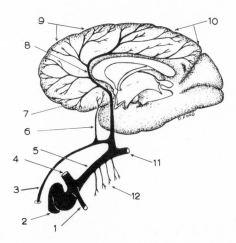

Fig. 63. A summary illustration of the distribution of the anterior cerebral artery. 1, proximal stem of posterior cerebral artery (posterior communicating artery); 2, internal carotid artery; 3, medial striate artery (Heubner-distal perforator); 4, middle cerebral artery; 5, anterior cerebral artery; 6, branch of medial striate artery to septal area; 7, orbital branches of anterior cerebral artery; 8, pericallosal stem of anterior cerebral artery; 9, frontal branches; 10, parietal branches; 11, anterior communicating artery; 12, proximal perforators to hypothalamus and preoptic area.

99

cerebral artery. Fig. 67 summarizes the distribution of the three cerebellar vessels.

1. Anastomotic connections are established ventrally through the Circle of Willis and also in the surface network of cortical vessels of both the cerebral and cerebellar hemispheres.

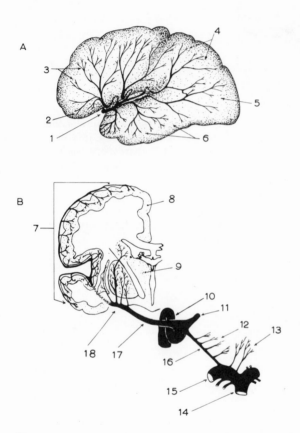

Fig. 64. A summary diagram of the distribution of the middle cerebral artery. Part A: 1, middle cerebral artery; 2, orbital branches; 3, frontal branches; 4, parietal branches; 5, occipital branches; 6, temporal branches. Part B illustrates the vessel distribution as viewed in a coronal plane to demonstrate the perforators; 7, cortical branches; 8, cerebral cortex; 9, diencephalon; 10, internal carotid artery; 11, stem of anterior cerebral artery; 12, diencephalic perforators arising from the proximal stem of the posterior cerebral artery (proximal perforators of the posterior cerebral cortex); 13, posteromedial (proximal) perforators from the mesencephalic stem of the posterior cerebral artery to the midbrain tegmentum; 14, basilar artery; 15, posterior cerebral artery; 16, proximal stem of the posterior cerebral artery; 17, middle cerebral artery; 18, lateral striate arteries (lenticulostriate or distal and proximal perforators of the middle cerebral artery).

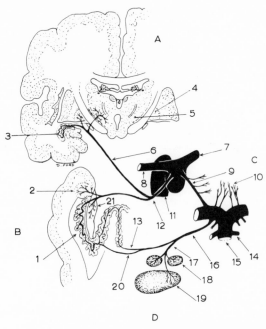

Fig. 65. A summary diagram illustrating the distribution of the anterior choroidal artery.
A, coronal section through the brain at the level of the ventrolateral thalamic nucleus;
B, horizontal section through the temporal lobe; C, arterial stem vessels; D, thalamus.
1, inferior horn of lateral ventricle with choroid plexus; 2, amygdala; 3, as 1; 4, medial
division of globus pallidus; 5, ventrolateral nucleus of thalamus; 6, choroid branch with
supply to medial pallidum and ventrolateral thalamus; 7, anterior cerebral artery;
8, middle cerebral artery; 9, proximal stem of posterior cerebral artery (posterior
communicating artery); 10, posteromedial (proximal) perforators of mesencephalic stem
of posterior cerebral artery to midbrain tegmentum; 11, internal carotid artery; 12, anterior
choroid artery; 13, branch from choroid diencephalic artery (posterior choroid) to choroid
plexus of third ventricle; 14, superior cerebellar artery; 15, basilar artery; 16, choroid-
diencephalic artery (distal perforator of the posterior cerebral artery); 17, branch to
geniculate bodies; 18, metathalamus (geniculate bodies); 19, caudal thalamus; 20, branch
of posterior choroid vessel to lateral ventricle; 21, parahippocampal gyrus.

D. Spinal cord.

1. Arterial supply (Fig. 68). The arterial support for the maintenance of
the spinal cord starts at the rostral end where two minor contributions are
made. Two small vessels arising from the vertebral artery fuse along the
ventral surface of the medulla and run caudally in the anterior median fissure
of the spinal cord as the anterior spinal artery (Fig. 54). Two other small
arteries, which arise from either the vertebral or posterior inferior cerebellar
arteries, run along the posterolateral margin of the cord and are interconnected
with each other at many levels. These are the posterior spinal arteries. It is

101

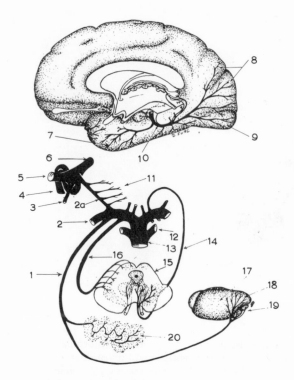

Fig. 66. A summary diagram of the distribution of the posterior cerebral artery. 1, choroid diencephalic artery to choroid plexus and thalamus (distal perforator); 2, posterior cerebral artery; 2a, proximal stem of posterior cerebral artery; 3, anterior choroid artery; 4, internal carotid artery; 5, middle cerebral artery; 6, anterior cerebral artery; 7, temporal branches; 8, parieto-occipital branches; 9, occipital branches; 10, posterior cerebral artery; 11, proximal perforators from proximal stem to ventral diencephalon; 12, superior cerebellar artery; 13, basilar artery; 14, posteromedial proximal perforators to midbrain tegmentum from the mesencephalic stem; 15, mesencephalon; 16, lateral nuclear and tectal branches from mesencephalic stem (distal perforators); 17, diencephalon; 18, pulvinar of thalamus; 19, geniculate bodies; 20, choroid plexus.

clear from the size of these vessels that they would be unable to supply the entire cord. Thus, to provide for an adequate blood supply throughout the cord there are extraspinal segmental arteries which enter through the intervertebral foramina and join the spinal arteries. These are the medullary arteries. There are 7 to 10 which join the anterior spinal artery and 6 to 8 which join the posterior spinal arteries. The largest of these occur at the upper lumbar spinal cord levels. An anterior vessel is called the great anterior medullary artery (artery of Adamkiewicz), while a similar posterior vessel is the great posterior medullary artery.

a. Surface network. Numerous vasa coronal vessels interconnect the posterior and anterior spinal arteries and form a dense plexus of small anastomotic vessels in the pia.

b. Intrinsic supply. Branches to the cord arise from both the posterior arterial plexus and the anterior spinal artery, as well as from the pial plexus. Rami arise at right-angles from the anterior spinal artery and enter the anterior median fissure, alternating to right or left to supply the ventral horn and adjacent white matter, and supplying roughly the anterior two-thirds of the cord. The posterior horns and adjacent white matter (posterior one-third of the cord) are supplied by numerous perforating vessels arising from the posterior arterial plexus.

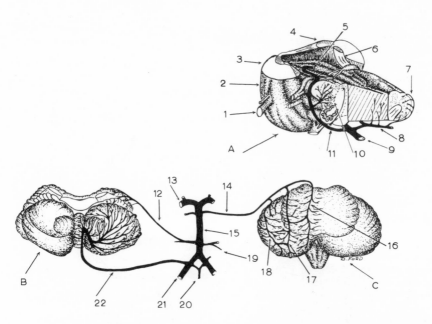

Fig. 67. A summary figure of the distribution of the arteries to the cerebellum. A, medulla-pons with left side cut away; B, ventral aspect of cerebellum; C, dorsal aspect of cerebellum. 1, trigeminal nerve; 2, pons; 3, middle cerebellar peduncle; 4, superior cerebellar peduncle; 5, posterior inferior cerebellar artery; 6, inferior peduncle; 7, vasa coronal vessels arising from anterior spinal artery; 8, anterior spinal artery supply to medulla; 9, vertebral artery; 10, branches of posterior inferior cerebellar artery to dorsolateral medulla (proximal perforators); 11, posterior inferior cerebellar artery; 12, anterior inferior cerebellar artery; 13, posterior cerebral artery; 14, superior cerebellar artery; 15, basilar artery; 16, pars medialis, superior cerebellar artery; 17, pars intermedia, superior cerebellar artery; 18, pars lateralis, superior cerebellar artery; 19, labyrinthine artery as a branch of the anterior inferior cerebellar artery (distal perforator); 20, anterior spinal artery; 21, vertebral artery; 22, posterior inferior cerebellar artery. Distal perforators of the posterior inferior and superior cerebellar arteries supply the deep nuclei of the cerebellum. Proximal perforators of the anterior inferior and superior cerebellar arteries appear directed to the basal pons and pontine tegmentum.

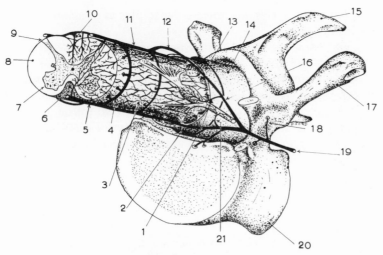

Fig. 68. Diagrammatic representation of the arterial supply to the spinal cord. 1, ganglionic branch from a posterior medullary artery; 2, anterior medullary artery; 3, pial arterial plexus; 4, arterial vasa corona; 5, anterior spinal artery; 6, central branch of anterior spinal artery; 7, anterior horn; 8, white matter of cord; 9, posterior horn; 10, central arterial branches from posterior spinal artery; 11, posterior spinal artery; 12, posterior medullary artery; 13, arachnoid; 14, dura mater; 15, spinal process; 16, posterior medullary artery; 17, transverse process; 18, osseous branch; 19, segmental artery from intercostal artery; 20, vertebral body; 21, radicular branch.

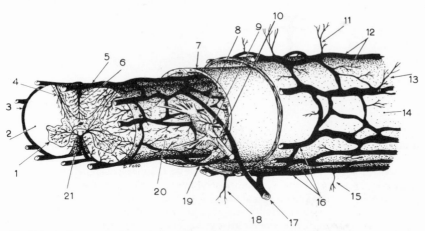

Fig. 69. A diagrammatic representation of the venous drainage of the spinal cord.
1, anterior horn; 2, white matter; 3, venous vasa corona; 4, posterior horn (with draining veins); 5, posterior medial spinal vein; 6, posterior central vein; 7, arachnoid; 8, posterior medullary vein; 9, ganglionic branch of posterior medullary vein; 10, radicular branch of posterior medullary vein; 11, osseous branch; 12, posterior epidural venous plexus; 13, osseous branch; 14, dura mater; 15, osseous branch; 16, anterior epidural plexus; 17, intervertebral vein; 18, basivertebral vein; 19, anterior medullary vein; 20, pial venous plexus; 21, sulcal vein.

104

c. Small radicular arteries arise from the segmental arteries for the anterior and posterior roots as well as for the dorsal root ganglion.

d. Surface anastomotic connections are established through the pial plexus.

2. Venous drainage. There is a rather plexiform arrangement for the surface veins of the cord in which an anterior longitudinal venous trunk and a series of posterior longitudinal vessels can be distinguished. These vessels are then interconnected to form a well-developed surface plexus into which the parenchymal vessels drain (Fig. 69). Drainage is such that the vessels draining the posterior half of the cord empty into the posterior medullary veins, while the anterior half drains into vessels which empty into the anterior medullary veins. The medial anterior part of the cord drains first into the anterior median spinal vein which in turn empties into the anterior medullary veins. The medullary veins finally empty into the veins of the external vertebral plexus, which in turn communicates with the inferior vena cava, azygos or hemiazygos vein, as well as with the sinuses of the dura mater. There is further a well-developed plexus of veins in the epidural space which also empties into the external vertebral plexus and which communicates with the veins of the spinal cord.

E. Blood-brain barrier. The concept that there is a barrier at the level of the brain capillaries which blocks the entry of many compounds into the CNS goes back to an observation by Ehrlich (1885) that certain aniline dyes, which stained all other tissues, failed to stain the brain.

1. Anatomically it would appear that the special organization of the brain capillaries would fit into a barrier concept. In the brain, capillary endothelial cells are interdigitated with each other and are completely invested by a well-developed basement membrane and finally by a layer of astrocyte glial foot processes which cover up to 85% of the capillary surface. Further, the endothelial cells are firmly and completely bonded to each other by "tight junctions". Thus, there is no large perivascular space in which pooling may occur, nor any areas of attenuation in the capillary wall which might facilitate movement of material out of the blood stream. This suggests that everything which enters into the brain parenchyma must pass through the walls of the endothelial cells and may probably also pass through the walls of the astrocytes as well before reaching the neurons. However, some material may reach the neurons by movement through the narrow extracellular spaces.

2. Whether a compound penetrates readily into the CNS, aside from anatomical factors, seems to depend on a variety of other factors.

a. Size of the molecule.

b. Degree of its dissociation.

c. Lipid solubility of the material.

d. Degree of binding to plasma proteins.

e. Presence or absence of specific transport systems.

f. Metabolic activity of the neurons.

g. Presence of enzymes in the capillary endothelium which may degrade the compound.

h. Presence of transport mechanisms within the cell membrane of the neuron which transports the compound out at a rate equal or at a rate only slightly less than the rate of entry, such as the sodium pump.

3. In general there appear to be three classes of molecule in relation to penetration of the blood-brain barrier.

a. Compounds which are essentially foreign to the brain such as various organic dyes, ferritin granules, horseradish peroxidase, etc., which are fairly large molecules and lack any specific role in CNS metabolism and which do not penetrate the brain parenchyma.

b. A large number of compounds whose entry depends on physical (or biochemical) constants such as lipid solubility, degree of dissociation, binding to plasma proteins, etc., which may then be observed to enter the brain at a rate influenced by these constants; for example, alcohol enters very readily as do steroid hormones.

c. Compounds for which there is a specific transport system into the brain, such as amino acids, RNA bases, etc. The degree of entry of these compounds may in turn be influenced by specific enzymes which degrade them on entry or which transport them back out. Many of these compounds have been shown to have very high levels of accumulation in neurons with essentially no accumulation in the surrounding neuropil.

F. Clinical considerations. In surveying a large number of brains at autopsy, it becomes clear very quickly that much of the pathology of the CNS is related to disease of the vascular system, some of which may be congenital, such as an arteriovenous malformation.

1. Arteriosclerosis. This is a condition which is marked by a loss of elasticity of the artery with thickening and hardening. Plaque formation in the walls reduces the lumen of the vessel and thus reduces the amount of blood reaching a given area of brain. Since the neurons are extremely dependent on a high pO_2, even a slight reduction of available oxygen (and glucose as well) may accelerate the normal loss of neurons with aging, causing a generalized atrophy of the brain from cerebral anemia. Cerebral anemia may also be associated with numerous systemic disorders leading to vascular insufficiency.

a. Small plaques may be dissected away from the wall of the vessel and be transported by the blood into some smaller vessel which then becomes occluded. This results in a loss of blood to some specific area of brain which

106

is thus infarcted and undergoes necrosis. Such areas are often seen in brains of older people as regions of encephalomalacia. These are regions which have undergone softening and necrosis subsequent to a loss of blood supply. The necrotic area becomes infiltrated with astrocyte processes which form a type of filmy scar traversing an irregular cystic cavity within the infarcted area. These are commonly seen in the basal ganglia and cerebral cortex, but no area of the CNS is immune to the development of such lesions. While these lesions are usually small they may be quite large and so located that, regardless of size, they produce specific neurological symptoms. The occurrence of encephalomalacia is increased in patients suffering from diabetes mellitus, as noted recently by Peress *et al.* This difference is apparent by the middle of the third decade and is maintained at all subsequent ages.

2. Aneurysms. These are focal widenings or sac-like dilatations in the wall of an artery due to congenital or arteriosclerotic defect. There may be fusiform dilations or berry-like projections. The wall of an aneurysm is weakened by the loss of the media and frequently by the absence of the internal elastic membrane. They are, therefore, regions of weakness in the arterial wall which may eventually rupture. If sufficiently large they may act as a space-occupying lesion by compression of adjacent CNS components. They may further become thrombotic. If the thrombosis projects into the vessel it will disrupt the blood supply to the area it serves.

3. Arteriovenous malformations. These occur where an artery empties directly into a vein rather than through a capillary bed. The result is that the area of brain normally supplied by that artery is by-passed, receives an inadequate blood supply and will atrophy. The vein into which the artery empties becomes greatly dilated and tortuous and may produce additional damage to the underlying soft CNS by compression. These malformations are also subject to hemorrhage.

4. Inflammatory reactions. In a variety of diseases there may be inflammation of the end arteries and small veins of the brain.
   a. Endarteritis. In this condition there is an inflammation of the intima of an artery which may be accompanied by collapse of the walls of the smaller vessels. This of course leads to infarction of the brain tissue normally supplied by this vessel.
   b. Phlebitis. In this condition the walls of the vein becomes infiltrated and there is the formation of a thrombus of clotted blood within the lumen. This serves to block the flow of blood from a given area of the brain and effectively interferes with its circulation.
   c. Meningitis. Inflammation of the meninges may also interfere with the vascular system by producing an inflammatory reaction within the intra-

meningeal vessels. Further, some investigators have suggested that the thin-walled veins may become compressed.

5. Strokes. This term refers to the sudden disruption of blood to a given area of brain. This may be caused by the sudden rupture of a vessel in a patient with hypertension, the occlusion of a CNS vessel by some thrombotic mass, or by occlusion of the internal carotid artery.

6. Traumatic injury may also damage blood vessels and lead to specific regions of degeneration.

a. Subdural hemorrhage. This is usually associated with trauma to the head wherein the veins become torn as they drain into the intradural venous sinuses (usually the superior sagittal sinus). The ensuing hemorrhage accumulates in the subdural space and compresses the underlying brain.

b. Epidural hemorrhage. This is relatively rare and seems primarily associated with skull fractures which lacerate the intradural vessels.

Chapter 9

VENTRICULAR SYSTEM

A. Formation. The ventricular system develops from the simple hollow neural tube which constitutes the early embryonic brain. As this tube expands rostro-dorsally to form the hemispheres, an extension of the hollow internal cavity projects out into the hemisphere to form the lateral ventricles. Both of these connect with the medially placed third ventricle via the intraventricular foramina of Monro. The segment of the tube between the two diencephalic masses becomes compressed mediolaterally to become the vertical slit of the third ventricle which is often bridged by a cellular mass between the two dorsal thalamic masses. This bridge is the massa intermedia (adhesio inter-thalamica). The hollow tubular cavity of the primitive brain is constricted in the midbrain to form the cerebral aqueduct. In the region of the pons-medulla the internal cavity flares out laterally during the time of the pontine flexure to form the fourth ventricle and at this point opens out into the external cerebrospinal fluid containing cavity (subarachnoid space) via the foramina of Luschka, or lateral apertures of the fourth ventricle, as well as through a posteromedial opening in the dorsum of the ventricle, the foramen of Magendie. The hollow central tubular cavity then becomes greatly con-stricted in the spinal cord to form the central canal (see Fig. 70).

1. At various places the roof of the ventricular system consists of only the ependymal lining of the primitive roof plate and the overlying pia mater. At these sites there is a vascular invasion to form the choroid plexuses in the lateral, third and fourth ventricles.

2. The lateral ventricle is a rather complex cavity which is related to each of the major portions of the hemisphere. It has been divided into anterior, inferior and posterior horns which relate to the frontal, temporal and occipital lobes, respectively. There is also a body which relates to some degree to the parietal lobe. The antrum is at the point of junction of the body, posterior and inferior horns.

3. The lateral ventricles are quite large during the early periods of develop-ment and become progressively constricted as the time of birth approaches. This constriction depends on myelinization of the various bundles of nerve fibers adjacent to it, and on the growth of nuclear masses of neurons which are along the walls of the system. In the process of decreasing the ventricular size, the posterior horn may be almost obliterated. It is thus of variable size in the adult.

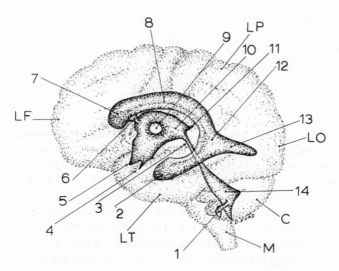

Fig. 70. A diagrammatic representation of the ventricular system of the brain in relation to the surface structures. 1, lateral recess of fourth ventricle (foramen of Luschka); 2, inferior horn of lateral ventricle; 3, cerebral aqueduct; 4, infundibular recess; 5, optic recess; 6, interventricular foramen (of Monro); 7, anterior horn of lateral ventricle; 8, central part (body) of lateral ventricle; 9, massa intermedia; 10, third ventricle; 11, pineal recess; 12, antrum of lateral ventricle; 13, posterior horn of lateral ventricle; 14, fourth ventricle; C, cerebellum; LF, frontal lobe; LO, occipital lobe; LP, parietal lobe; LT, temporal lobe; M, medulla oblongata.

4. The cavities of the ventricular system are lined by ependymal cells, whose free surfaces possess both microvilli and cilia.

a. Ventricular surface of the epithelium is ciliated. The pattern of ciliary beat suggests that it aids the flow of cerebrospinal fluid from the lateral to the third ventricle and then down the cerebral aqueduct to escape from the ventricular cavities through the foramina of Luschka.

b. Cells beneath the posterior commissure are modified to form a pseudo-stratified epithelium, the subcommissural organ, which appears to be secretory in several subprimate mammals.

B. Cerebrospinal fluid (CSF). The ventricular system is filled with the CSF, which is a clear, almost cell-free, fluid. It is slightly more acid than arterial plasma, having a pH of 7.3, while the plasma averages 7.4. It normally contains very little protein (15—45 mg%) which varies from individual to individual and with age (10—20 mg% in children and around 40 mg% in adults). It also contains small amounts of amino acids, sugar, calcium, potassium, sodium, chloride, magnesium, iodine, lactate, lactate dehydrogenase, creatinine, uric acid, urea and cholesterol. Traces of ^{131}I-triiodothyronine have been found in the CSF after intravenous injection of the hormone, suggesting some move-

110

ment of the hormone into the CSF either through the choroid plexus or through the brain parenchyma. A few cells (mostly lymphoid elements) are also usually seen (5/μl).

1. Protein increases in the CSF in certain clinical conditions (syphilis, multiple sclerosis, tumors, polyradiculitis).
   a. Pandy test. Positive with elevation of either total protein or gamma-globulin. (Normal spinal fluid gamma-globulin should not exceed 13% of the total protein content. Gamma-globulin is elevated in both neurosyphilis and multiple sclerosis.)

2. CSF glucose is normally about 60—80 mg%.

3. CSF chlorides are normally about 700—750 mg% and reduced in tuberculous meningitis to as low as 500—600 mg%.

4. The presence of large numbers of cellular elements in the CSF is usually associated with subarachnoid hemorrhage as from a ruptured aneurysm which may produce up to 150 000 erythrocytes/ml. Intraparenchymal hemorrhage from hypertension or trauma seldom causes as large a rise in cell count unless the hemorrhage dissects its way out and into the subarachnoid space or into the ventricular system. Traumatic spinal taps may also give rise to bloody samples of CSF. Large numbers of leucocytes may be anticipated in inflammatory disease affecting the leptomeninges.

5. Pressure. Maximal normal pressures of CSF recorded at the cisterna magna are about 150 ml of saline, though some normals have been recorded as high as 180 ml saline. Pressure measurements taken at the lumbar sac with the subject sitting upright may be as high as 397 ml of saline. While in the recumbent position, the pressure from the lumbar sac is about 150 ml of saline, comparable to that obtained from the cisterna magna. Pressure of the CSF is readily elevated by coughing or sneezing.
   a. The Queckenstedt test. This test is performed by compressing the jugular veins during lumbar puncture. Normally there is a prompt rise in CSF pressure which is maintained as long as the veins are compressed. Compression of only one vein causes a moderate rise in pressure. If CSF pressure fails to rise or fall promptly, a block in the CSF system may be suspected between the site of puncture and site of venous compression. Absence of a rise in pressure could be due to thrombosis of the jugular vein. The test should not be performed if a cerebral tumor or bleeding is suspected.

6. Formation. The CSF is formed largely by the choroid plexuses as a process of active secretion of a hypertonic solution in relation to sodium which is brought to isotonicity within the ventricular cavity by diffusion of

111

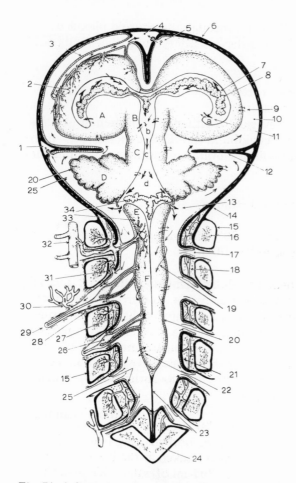

Fig. 71. A diagrammatic scheme indicating the various sources of formation of the cerebrospinal fluid and the sites of resorption. A, telencephalon; B, diencephalon; C, mesencephalon; D, cerebellum; E, myelencephalon; F, spinal cord; a, lateral ventricle; b, third ventricle; c, cerebral aqueduct; d, fourth ventricle. 1, transverse sinus with arachnoid granulation; 2, CSF resorption into pial plexus; 3, superior cerebral vein; 4, superior sagittal sinus; 5, arachnoid granulation; 6, dura mater; 7, lateral ventricle; 8, choroid plexus; 9, exchange of fluid between brain parenchyma and subarachnoid space; 10, subarachnoid space; 11, exchange of fluid between brain parenchyma and intra-ventricular fluid; 12, tentorium cerebelli; 13, CSF exiting through foramen of Luschka; 14, point of junction between dura mater spinalis and periostal dura at foramen magnum; 15, vertebral periosteum; 16, vertebra; 17, intervertebral foramen; 18, epidural space; 19, arrow indicating CSF flow down over dorsum of spinal cord; 20, pia mater; 21, dura mater; 22, fluid exchange across pial-glial membrane; 23, filum terminale; 24, os coccygis; 25, arachnoid; 26, spinal ganglion; 27, epidural space; 28, dural sheath of spinal nerve blending with epineurium distal to ganglion; 29, perineuronal space of spinal nerve; 30, lymphatic plexus draining perineuronal space; 31, arachnoid granulation in epidural vein; 32, external vertebral venous plexus; 33, CSF entering pial plexus; 34, choroid plexus of fourth ventricle.

water across the ependymal lining of the ventricular surface. The rate of formation seems to be accelerated by elevations in blood pressure.

a. Ideas on the rate of formation have varied considerably. Figures derived by Sweet *et al.* (1954) suggest that it ranges from 50 to 150 ml/day, though others give much larger rates.

7. Volume of CSF. In man the total volume of CSF is about 140 ml of which about 23 ml is in the ventricular cavities.

8. Flow. The direction of CSF flow is from the lateral ventricles (where the greatest volume is formed) through the interventricular foramina of Monro into the third ventricle and down the cerebral aqueduct into the fourth ventricle where it escapes into the subarachnoid spaces by passing through the lateral foramen of Luschka and the posteromedial foramen of Magendie. Flow is presumably facilitated by the beating of ependymal cilia. Once out in the subarachnoid spaces the fluid diffuses over the surface of the brain.

a. Resorption. Resorption of CSF into the venous drainage occurs primarily at the arachnoid granulations, where the rate of resorption varies directly with CSF pressure. Most of these granulations are associated with the superior sagittal sinus, though such granulations have been seen to occur in relation to all intradural venous sinuses. By electron microscopy, these granulations appear to be made up of columns of cells through which run channels perpendicular to the free surface of the granulation which is capped by an epithelial layer. Experimentally, when CSF pressure is high these channels appear straight and open. When CSF pressure is low, these channels are folded up and presumably closed. Thus, they seem as valves which may permit flow of CSF into the various sinuses when open. How the fluid passes through the cells of the epithelial cap remains uncertain, though passive diffusion has been suggested. Some CSF has also been observed to drain out through the pia-arachnoid cuffs at the bony foraminal exits of the spinal and cranial nerves, into the perineuronal spaces which are in turn drained by the lymphatic system. There is, in addition, evidence to support some resorption of solutes contained in the CSF into the small vessels of the pia mater. Finally, there seems to be some degree of fluid exchange along all membrane-covered surfaces of the brain (Fig. 71).

b. Function. The CSF has usually been stated to protect the brain from sudden shocks from the outside. A wide variety of studies also suggest that at least the ventricular CSF may serve to remove waste products of neuronal and glial metabolism by the sink action of the ventricular CSF which has extremely low concentrations of many solutes relative to the brain.

C. Clinical consideration of the ventricular system.

1. Hydrocephalus. Indicates an excess of CSF which could be due to either an over-production or under-resorption.

a. Cerebral dysgenesis. In many types of cerebral malformation there is a failure of development of some part of the brain with an accumulation of CSF to compensate for the absent brain tissue.

b. Excessive production of CSF is rare, but may be caused by a papilloma of the choroid plexus (readily treated by surgical removal of the papilloma).

c. Obstruction to the flow of CSF is probably responsible for most cases of hydrocephalus. It may occur at any level.

(i) Atretic occlusion of the cerebral aqueduct causes dilation of the rostrally placed components of the ventricular system.

(ii) A single foramen of Monro may be occluded as by a cyst, causing a unilateral ventricular dilation.

(iii) Meningeal inflammatory disease is often accompanied by occlusion of the lateral foramen of Luschka with the consequent dilation of the entire ventricular system.

(iv) Deficiency of resorption of CSF may occur following meningitis due to obstruction of the arachnoid granulations. It may also occur following subarachnoid hemorrhage or if the CSF protein content is too high.

(v) Hydrocephalus ex vacuo. This term refers to the excessive volume of CSF observed in the subarachnoid space and in the ventricular cavities as a result of cerebral atrophy.

Chapter 10

CNS PATHWAYS

A. The various levels of the CNS are interconnected with each other by numerous short and long ascending and descending fiber bundles. Thus, there are the short nerve fiber links which link different levels of the spinal cord together which run in the fasciculus proprius adjacent to the grey matter of the cord; longer nerve bundles which project afferent signals entering from the periphery to higher levels for complex reflex responses or for final recognition by the cerebral cortex; long descending projection systems which transmit information from the cerebral cortex to motor cells to initiate motor responses, plus numerous loop systems such as those which unite the limbic system to the hypothalamic autonomic system or the cerebellum to the motor system. Our understanding of how these interconnections are made has been accumulating since the late nineteenth century.

Briefly, some of the methods which have been used to provide information as to the specific location of various tracts conveying specific types of information are as follows.

1. The study of myelinogenesis was introduced by Flechsig and makes use of the fact that various tracts myelinate at different times during embryonic life.

2. The impregnation of nerve cell bodies and their processes with gold and silver salts was introduced by Golgi. While it provided some information in general as to where fibers went, it was often difficult to determine where the fibers ended.

3. By far the greatest information has come from the study of pathological nerve preparations wherein a fiber bundle was sectioned or damaged accidently and the course of the degenerating antegrade nerve fibers determined by various histological procedures.

a. Gudden's method. In about 1870 Gudden discovered that if one injured the cortex of a newborn rabbit and then examined the brain 7—8 weeks later, the fiber systems originating from that region of cortex had atrophied or been resorbed and that the nuclei on which the fibers terminated were diminished in size. The degree of wasting was much less in adult animals and could be discerned only after a longer period of degeneration.

b. Marchi's method. This procedure, which was described in about 1890, depended on the fact that the degenerating myelin in the distal portion of a sectioned or damaged nerve could be impregnated with osmium following mordanting with potassium bichromate. The changes in the myelin require about 10—20 days to reach a maximum degree after injury at which time the myelin appears as black dots or cylindrical particles.

c. More recently Nauta and Gygax (1954) and Nauta (1957) have worked out a silver impregnation method which successfully demonstrates fine degenerating axons (not the myelin) which appears black against a yellow background. Fine degenerating fibers may also be observed using the method of Glees (1946). This procedure also impregnates the terminal boutons, but does not distinguish between normal and degenerating terminals. Degenerating boutons may also be discerned with the Nauta technique.

d. The Fink-Heimer impregnation procedure (1966—1967) is perhaps the latest to be used with degenerating axons and shows the distribution of extremely fine unmyelinated degenerating fibers.

4. Nissl stains may be used to study the retrograde changes occurring in the nerve cell bodies, wherein one gets varying degrees of chromatolysis, swelling, eosinophilia and a shift of the nucleus to the periphery (Fig. 72).

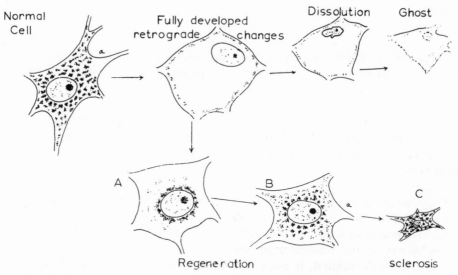

Fig. 72. A diagrammatic illustration of the changes which occur in a neuron during retrograde degeneration and which lead to cloudy swelling and dissolution of the Nissl substance and finally the formation of a ghost which will itself disappear. Regenerative changes are indicated at A and B wherein the new Nissl substance is first seen in the cytoplasm as a perinuclear halo and then slowly extends out into the cell (B) to resume a normal appearance. However, if the regenerating axon of this cell does not establish a connection with a receptor or an effector, the cell will undergo a condensation (sclerosis) and die, as in C.

116

Dissolution of the cell continues until only a vague cell outline or ghost remains. Not all cells may show these changes, however. One may also observe the recovery phases in neurons that do not die from the injury. New basophilic material appears first around the nucleolus and then around the nucleus (Fig. 72A). Those which successfully send out new sprouts and attain a final connection with a receptor or effector will mature into normal neurons (Fig. 72B). If this final association is not achieved, the cell will finally undergo late atrophy (Fig. 72C) even though it recovered from the original injury. According to Bodian (1947), it takes about two weeks for the ventral horn motor neurons of a monkey to start to show regenerative changes which finally are nearly complete in 80 days, though it may take up to six months for complete regeneration.

5. Transneuronal degenerative changes have been observed in a series of nuclei following damage to their primary afferent supply. The changes which occur can be observed with a Nissl stain and consist of changes in cell, nuclear and nucleolar size and in the neuronal population density of the denervated nucleus. Such changes have been observed in the cochlear nuclei of cats, lateral geniculate bodies of monkeys, cats and rabbits and in the olive and cerebellum in a number of species including man. Eventually the cells may undergo total atrophy and disappear.

6. There are also physiological procedures for following tract systems by recording evoked potential initiated by various stimuli. More recently it has become possible to record the action potentials of single cells or fibers (single unit recording).

B. Organization. Fig. 73 illustrates a few of the ways in which the various levels of the CNS may be linked together to utilize the responses which may result from cutaneous stimuli of pain or temperature from the body. It demonstrates the multiplicity of levels at which interaction may occur to produce a reflex response or conscious awareness of the stimulus. It is to be understood that this does not apply for all types of sensory information, etc. Further, no attempt has been made to indicate whether or not the various projections ascend ipsilaterally or contralaterally.

One may start at the receptor for pain and temperature. The cell bodies for these receptors are found in the dorsal root ganglia (drg) at "a" (Fig. 73). The proximal fiber may synapse on a cell in the dorsal horn (d) at the level of entry or one or two segments rostral or caudal from this point. Several levels of neural interaction may then result from this input, starting at the level of input (1) and extending up to the level of the neothalamus (nth) and cortex (6).

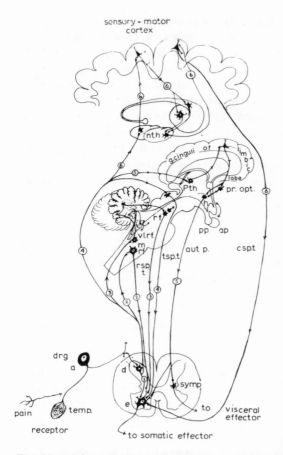

Fig. 73. A schematic illustration of the various suprasegmental levels of interaction which may result from a single stimulation of a pain or temperature receptor. (See text for further details.)

1. Reflex connections are made on motor cells (e) at this level for a local segmental response. These connections may be ipsi-, contra- or bilateral.

2. An ascending component (2) synapses on cells of the medial reticular formation (mrf) of the medulla from which arise descending projection fibers which pass into the cord via one of the reticulospinal tracts (rspt) to terminate finally on effector (e) motor neurons in the ventral horn. (These and the subsequent connections on the ventral motor neurons are probably all mediated via internuncial cells.)

3. Other ascending projections related to pain and temperature terminate in the ventrolateral reticular formation (vl.rf.) of the medulla. This nucleus

118

relays the information to the cerebellar cortex via mossy fibers which terminate on granule cells which in turn synapse on the Purkinje cells. Purkinje cells of the cortex project their axons to the deep cerebellar nuclei which then relay the signal to the reticular formation of the midbrain (also to the red nucleus and ventral lateral nucleus of the thalamus). The midbrain reticular formation then provides its own contribution to the reticulospinal tract projection. There may also be rubrospinal tract projections down to the final effector elements. Some fibers also project rostrally from the reticular formation to terminate in the thalamus.

4. The fourth ascending projection terminates in the superior colliculus of the midbrain from which arises the crossed tectospinal tract (tsp. t), which again activates the effector elements.

5. The thalamus receives the information at two levels, one a phylogenetically old one, the so-called primitive thalamic nuclei (pth). These consist of the nuclei of the internal and external medullary laminae and of the midline nuclei. The nuclei project rather nonspecifically to the limbic cortex of the gyrus cinguli. From here the signal is relayed to the preoptic area (pr. opt.) for relay to the hypothalamus or directly to the hypothalamus (h). Finally, the hypothalamic structures project, possibly by a multisynaptic autonomic pathway (aut. p.), to the preganglionic nuclei of parasympathetic cranial nerves or to the intermediolateral cell column of the spinal cord to synapse on sympathetic (symp) preganglionic motor neurons.

6. The other projection into the thalamus is to neothalamic nuclei (nth) such as the ventroposterolateral nucleus which relays the information to the postcentral gyrus of the cerebral cortex in a highly topographic manner. From here the information is projected to the caudate nucleus and putamen of the corpus striatum by the pyramidal cells of layer 5. The cells of the striatum in turn relay the signal directly to the motor cortex of the precentral gyrus and premotor area or via a relay in the ventrolateral and ventral anterior nuclei of the thalamus. Finally, the motor and premotor neurons of layer 5 form the large descending motor projection system, which exits from the cerebral hemisphere through the internal capsule and finally attains the level of the motor cells of the spinal cord after passing down through the lateral and anterior corticospinal tracts (csp. t). A corticobulbar projection serves to activate motor cells of the cranial nerves.

What has been described is a series of suprasegmental levels which are to a considerable extent integrated with each other. Similar sorts of interconnections could be diagrammed for the trigeminal nerve pain-temperature components.

Chapter 11

SENSORY SYSTEMS

A. Pain, temperature and light touch (includes itch, tickle and erotic sensations). These particular sensations from the body can be considered together, not only because of a sharing of a common ascending path in the anterolateral fasciculus (spinothalamic tracts + spinoreticular and spinotectal tracts) but because the sensations are poorly localized at the periphery and provide for an input at various suprasegmental levels including two at the level of the thalamus. A large proportion of the afferent information enters the paleothalamic nuclei of the midline and intralaminar nuclear group and is then relayed rather nonspecifically to the limbic cortex of the gyrus cinguli. Some fibers pass through the centromedial nucleus (centrum medianum) to terminate in the nucleus centralis lateralis, while some investigators believe there is a significant contribution to the centromedial nucleus. The remaining fibers terminate in the ventroposterolateral nucleus of the thalamus in a topographically specific manner. Neurons of this nucleus then relay the information to the postcentral gyrus, again in a topographically specific manner. These sensations may be considered as primitive in relation to such tactile senses as two-point discrimination, vibratory and position sense.

1. The various levels of interaction for this system are illustrated in Fig. 74. It is to be noted that the sensory input establishes connections for reflex response in the dorsal horn of the spinal cord where an interaction with ventral horn motor neurons may occur. Further suprasegmental levels of interaction occur in the medulla in the medial reticular formation (MRF) which then gives rise to one portion of the reticulospinal tract. Another medullary interaction is with cells of the lateral reticular formation (LRF) which relays the signal to the cerebellum. Some sensory input then continues rostrally, establishing contacts on cells of the central grey and superior colliculus of the midbrain and finally in the nucleus centralis lateralis and other intralaminal thalamic nuclei as well as on the ventroposterolateral nucleus of the thalamus.

a. The ascending course of this pathway may also be appreciated by attempting to locate the position of the ascending tract in relation to the various nuclei where interactions occur by using Pal-Weigert preparations. A convenient way to attempt this is to mount half a picture of a Pal-Weigert preparation on a mounting board, then diagram the mirror image of the figure alongside it. Do this for each of the levels at which significant interactions of the particular tract being studied occur. An example of how such a mapping of tracts in relation to Pal-Weigert preparations would appear is illustrated in Figs 75—79. (Note that anterolateral fasciculus = spinal lemniscus in brain stem.)

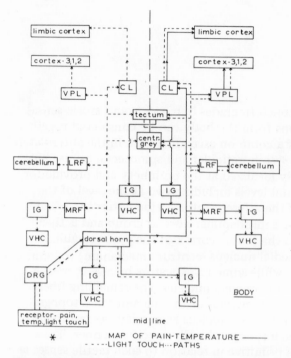

MAP OF PAIN-TEMPERATURE ———
- - - - - LIGHT TOUCH - - - PATHS

Fig. 74. A schematic representation of the various units of the nervous system involved in the projection of sensations of pain, temperature and light touch (+ itch, tickle and erotic sensations) from the periphery into the CNS to establish reflex connections at a number of suprasegmental levels. This illustration is only for the body. centr. grey, central grey of midbrain; CL, nucleus centralis lateralis thalami (centrolateral nucleus); DRG, dorsal root ganglion cells; IG, intermediate grey of the spinal cord; LRF, lateral reticular formation of the medulla; MRF, medial reticular formation of the medulla; VHC, ventral horn motor neuron; VPL, ventroposterolateral nucleus of thalamus.

Fig. 75. An illustration of the distribution of cells in the spinal cord and their fibers which are related to transmission of pain, temperature and light touch (upper thoracic cord). df, dorsal funiculus; dh, dorsal horn; drg, dorsal root ganglion; fc, fasciculus cuneatus; fg, fasciculus gracilis; ig, intermediate grey of spinal cord; ilh, intermediolateral horn (autonomic); lf, lateral funiculus; ls, lumbrosacral fibers; npd, nucleus proprius dorsalis; pm, posteromarginal nucleus; p.t. + lt., pain, temperature, light touch; sg, substantia gelatinosa; t, thoracic fibers; vh, ventral horn; vf, ventral funiculus (anterior).

Fig. 76. An illustration of the distribution of cells and fiber tracts at the level of the medulla concerned with the transmission of pain, temperature and light touch (p.t. + lt) from the body. a, arcuate nucleus; c, cervical fibers; dlrf, dorsolateral reticular formation; inf cbl pd, inferior cerebellar peduncle; inf ol, inferior olive; inf v, inferior vestibular nucleus; ml, medial lemniscus; mlf, medial longitudinal fasciculus; mrf, medial reticular formation; mv, medial vestibular nucleus; nV, descending nucleus of trigeminal nerve; py, pyramid; s, sacral fibers; t, thoracic fibers; ts, tract of the nucleus solitarius; t sp t, tectospinal tract; XII, hypoglossal nerve nucleus.

122

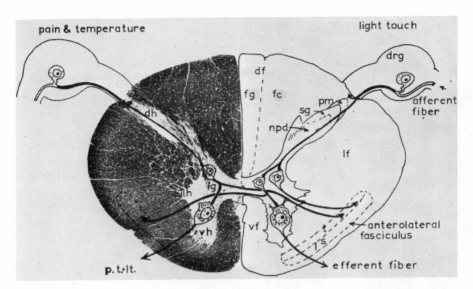

Fig. 75

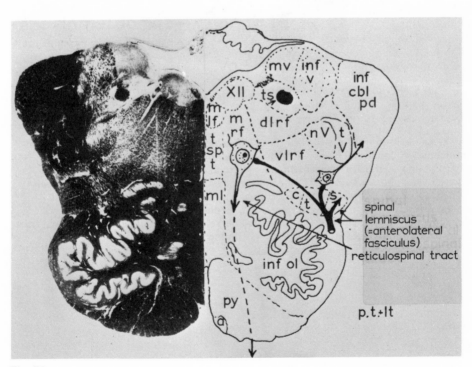

Fig. 76

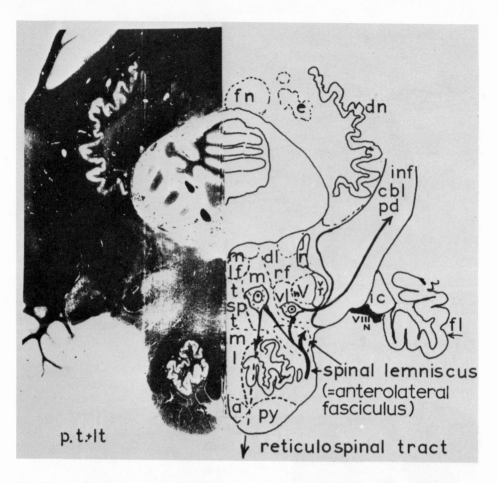

Fig. 77. An illustration of the distribution of neurons and fiber tracts at the level of the pontomedullary junction concerned with pain, temperature and light touch from the body (p.t. + lt). a, arcuate nucleus; dlrf, dorsolateral reticular formation; dn, dentate nucleus; e, emboliform nucleus; fl, flocculus; fn, fastigial nucleus; ic, inferior cochlear nucleus; inf cbl pd, inferior cerebellar peduncle; jr, juxtarestiform body; m, medial reticular formation; ml, medial lemniscus; mlf, medial longitudinal fasciculus; nV-vT, descending nucleus and tract of the trigeminal nerve; py, pyramid; t sp t, tectospinal tract; vl, ventrolateral reticular formation; VIII, vestibulocochlear nerve root.

124

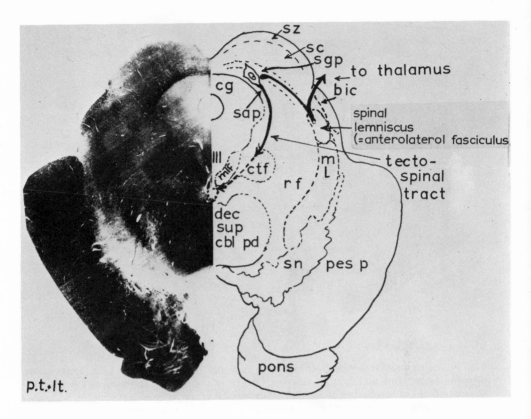

Fig. 78. An illustration of the distribution of neurons and fiber tracts at the level of the superior colliculus concerned with pain, temperature and light touch (p.t. lt.) from the body. bic, brachium of the inferior colliculus; cg, central grey; ctf, central tegmental fasciculus; dec sup cbl pd, decussation of the superior cerebellar peduncle; ml, medial lemniscus; mlf, medial longitudinal fasciculus; pes p, pes pedunculi; rf, reticular formation; sap, stratum album profundum; sc, superior colliculus; sn, substantia nigra; sgp, stratum griseum profundum; sz, stratum zonale; III, nucleus of oculomotor nerve.

125

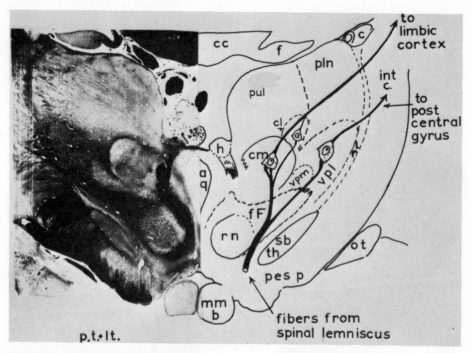

Fig. 79. An illustration of the distribution of cells and fibers concerned with transmission of pain, temperature and light touch (p.t. + lt.) from the body at the level of the thalamus. aq, rostral end of cerebral aqueduct; c, caudate nucleus; cc, corpus callosum; cl, nucleus centralis lateralis; cm, centrum medianum; f, fornix; fF, field of Forel; h, habenular nucleus; int c, internal capsule; lr, lateral reticular formation; mmb, mammillary bodies; ot, optic tract; pes p, pes pedunculi; rn, red nucleus; sb th, subthalamic nucleus; vpl, ventroposterolateral nucleus of thalamus; vpm, ventroposteromedial nucleus of thalamus. Note indication of terminals in both cm and cl of primitive intralaminar thalamic nuclear complex.

Fig. 80. A schematic diagram of the various nuclear areas within the CNS concerned with transmission of pain, temperature and light touch (p.t. + lt) from the face from the receptors to the cortex. CG, central grey of midbrain; CL, nucleus centralis lateralis of thalamus; DLRF, dorsolateral reticular formation; IG, intermediate grey matter; main sens. V, main sensory nucleus of trigeminal nerve; mes. nuc. V, mesencephalic nucleus of trigeminal nerve; motor V, motor nucleus of trigeminal nerve; MRF, medial reticular formation; spinal nuc V, descending spinal nucleus of trigeminal nerve; VHC, ventral horn motor neuron; VLRF, ventrolateral reticular formation; VPM, ventroposteromedial nucleus of thalamus.

Fig. 81. An illustration of the distribution of cells and fibers concerned with pain, temperature and light touch (p.t. + lt.) from the face at the level of entry of the trigeminal nerve in the midpontine region. ctf, central tegmental fasciculus; l. lemn., lateral lemniscus; m cbl pd, middle cerebellar peduncle (brachium pontis); mes tr V + nuc, mesencephalic tract and nucleus of the trigeminal nerve; ml, medial lemniscus; mlf, medial longitudinal fasciculus; s cbl pd, superior cerebellar peduncle (brachium conjunctivum); Tr. g, trigeminal ganglion.

126

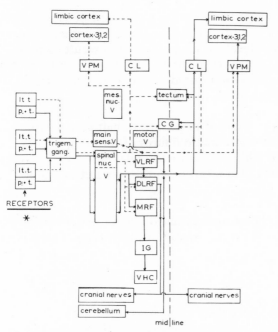

MAP OF TRIGEMINAL PAIN & TEMPERATURE PATHWAYS ——
LIGHT TOUCH PATHWAY ------

Fig. 80

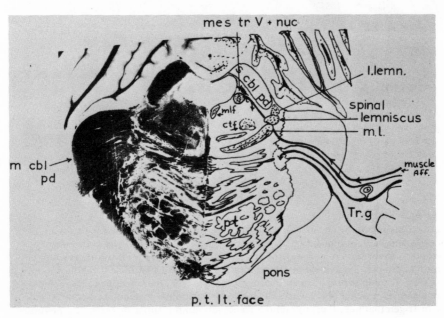

Fig. 81

2. Pain, temperature, light touch, etc., sensations from the face (Fig. 80) establish comparable connections as do those arising from the body. Again, there are numerous suprasegmental levels of interaction with resulting reflex components being activated to produce responses in somatic or visceral motor nuclei. In this instance motor neurons are located in cranial nerve motor nuclei as well as in the ventral horns of the spinal cord.

a. As in the previous section a series of mock-ups of half photographs of Pal-Weigert preparations and half diagrammatic figures of the components and tract positions can be created which illustrate the position of the descending and ascending units associated with pain (etc.) from the face until attaining the highest level of interaction (Figs 81—87).

B. Discriminative sensations (two-point discrimination, vibratory sense, conscious awareness of body position (proprioception) and stereognosis) from

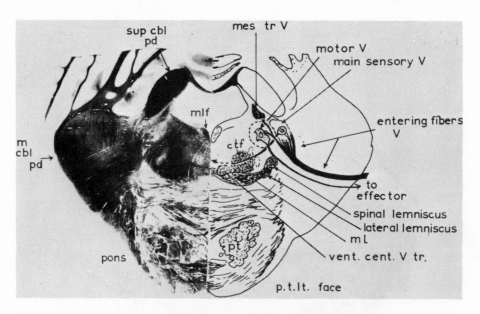

Fig. 82. An illustration of the distribution of cells and fibers concerned with pain, temperature and light touch (p.t. + lt.) from the face at the level of the main sensory nucleus and of the motor nucleus of the trigeminal nerve in the midpontine region. ctf, central tegmental fasciculus; m cbl pd, middle cerebellar peduncle (brachium pontis); main sensory V, main sensory trigeminal nucleus; mes tr V, mesencephalic tract of trigeminal nerve; ml, medial lemniscus; mlf, medial longitudinal fasciculus; motor V, motor nucleus of trigeminal nerve; pt, pyramidal tract; sup cbl pd, superior cerebellar peduncle (brachium conjunctivum); vent. cent. V tr., ventral central trigeminal tract.

128

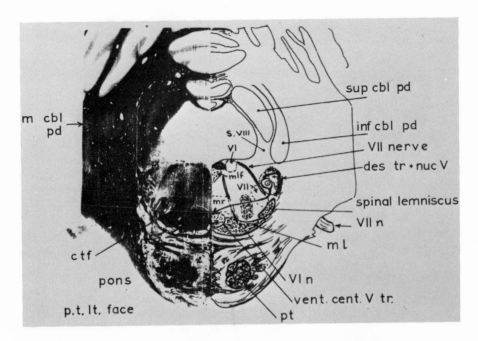

Fig. 83. An illustration of the distribution of cells and fibers concerned with pain, temperature and light touch (p.t. + lt.) from the face at the level of the caudal pons. ctf, central tegmental fasciculus; des tr + nuc V, descending trigeminal tract and nucleus; inf cbl pd, inferior cerebellar peduncle (restiform body); m cbl pd, middle cerebellar peduncle (brachium pontis); ml, medial lemniscus; mlf, medial longitudinal fasciculus; mr, medial reticular formation; pt, pyramidal tract; sup cbl pd, superior cerebellar peduncle (brachium conjunctivum); vent. cent. V tr., ventral central trigeminal tract; VIn, nucleus of abducens nerve; VIIn, nucleus of facial nerve; S. VIII, superior nucleus of the vestibular nerve.

the body. These particular modalities of sensation share a common tract system. They are often termed the dorsal column sensations, inasmuch as they ascend to higher centers in the dorsal funiculus of the spinal cord. This pathway may be illustrated schematically as indicated in Fig. 88.

1. Note that the sensory input entering via the dorsal root fibers of the dorsal root ganglion may elicit ipsi- or contralateral reflex responses at the level of entry or be propagated to higher levels wherein the stimulus information is relayed by the gracilis and cuneate nuclei of the medulla to the thalamus and thence to the primary sensory cortex of the postcentral gyrus and the paracentral lobule (areas 3, 1 and 2 according to Brodmann; sensory area I). Note also that there are corticofugal fibers which parallel the path of the sensory input which terminate on the relay cells in the cuneate and gracilis nuclei. The precise function of these corticocuneate and gracile projections

129

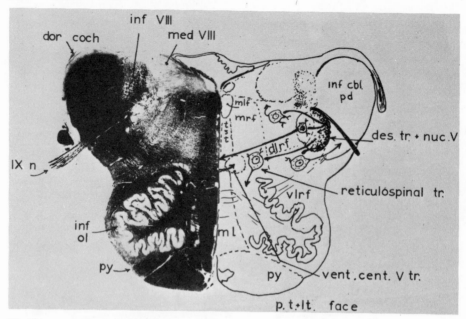

Fig. 84

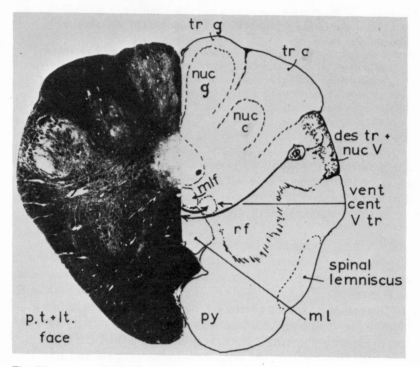

Fig. 85

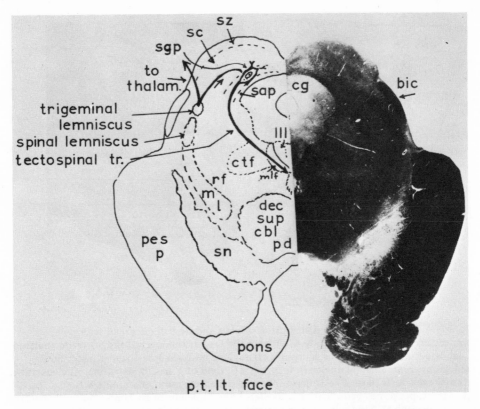

Fig. 86. An illustration of the distribution of cells and fibers concerned with pain, temperature and light touch (p.t. + lt.) from the face at the level of the superior colliculus. bic, brachium of inferior colliculus; cg, central grey of midbrain; ctf, central tegmental fasciculus; dec sup cbl pd, decussation of superior cerebellar peduncle; ml, medial lemniscus; mlf, medial longitudinal fasciculus; pes p, pes pedunculi; rf, reticular formation; sn, substantia nigra; sap, stratum album profundum; sc, superior colliculus (referring to total area); sgp, stratum griseum profundum; sz, stratum zonale; III, oculomotor nucleus.

Fig. 84. An illustration of the distribution of cells and fibers concerned with pain, temperature and light touch (p.t. + lt.) from the face at the level of the rostral medulla. des. tr. + nuc. V, descending trigeminal tract and nucleus; dlrf, dorsolateral reticular formation; dor coch, dorsal cochlear nucleus; inf cbl pd, inferior cerebellar peduncle (restiform body); inf ol, inferior olive; inf VIII, inferior vestibular nucleus; med VIII, medial vestibular nucleus; ml, medial lemniscus; mlf, medial longitudinal fasciculus; mrf, medial reticular formation; py, pyramid; tst, tectospinal tract; vlrf, ventrolateral reticular formation; IXn, nerve fibers of the glossopharyngeal nerve.

Fig. 85. An illustration of the distribution of cells and fibers concerned with pain, temperature and light touch (p.t. + lt.) from the face at the level of the caudal closed part of the medulla. des tr + nuc V, descending trigeminal tract and nucleus; ml, medial lemniscus; mlf, medial longitudinal fasciculus; nuc c, nucleus cuneatus; nuc g, nucleus gracilis; py, pyramid; rf, reticular formation; tr c, fasciculus cuneatus; tr g, fasciculus gracilis; vent cent V tr, ventral central trigeminal tract.

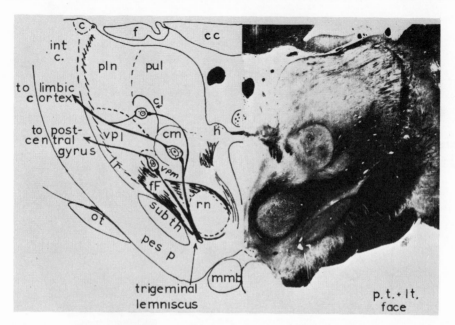

Fig. 87. An illustration of the distribution of cells and fibers concerned with pain, temperature and light touch (p.t. + lt.) from the face at the level of the posterior thalamus. c, caudate nucleus; cc, corpus callosum; cl, nucleus centralis lateralis; cm, centrum medianum (centromedial nucleus); f, fornix; fF, field of Forel; h, habenular nucleus; int c, internal capsule; lr, lateral reticular nucleus of thalamus; mmb, mammillary bodies; ot, optic tract; pes p, pes pedunculi; pln, posterolateral nucleus of thalamus; pul, pulvinar; rn, red nucleus; sub th, subthalamic nucleus; vpl, ventroposterolateral nucleus of thalamus; vpm, ventroposteromedial nucleus of thalamus. Note indication of terminals in both cm and cl of primitive intralaminar thalamic nuclear complex.

remains uncertain, but they appear to have an inhibitory effect on the activity of the neurons of these nuclei and may in some way serve to sharpen perception. Some facilitation of the activity of these neurons is also known to occur.

a. This projection to the cortex demonstrates a somatotopic distribution (see various standard texts of neuroanatomy for diagrams depicting the relative areas of sensory distribution to the postcentral gyrus). The distribution of the relay neurons in the ventroposterolateral nucleus of the thalamus also shows a somatotopic localization.

b. It should be further pointed out that the distribution of sensory information is not restricted to the postcentral gyrus, but extends onto the adjacent precentral gyrus and down into the lateral fissure along the inferior aspect of the opercular cortex to the insula (sensory area II). This region along the upper edge of the lateral fissure adjacent to the insula is referred to as the second somatosensory area, which is considerably smaller and less specifically organized than sensory area I.

132

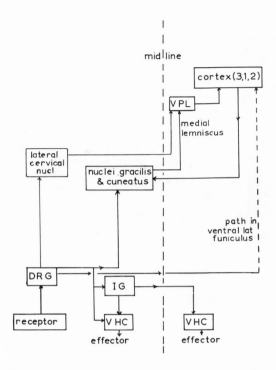

Fig. 88. A schematic illustration of the connections involved in the perception of fine discriminative sensations from the body from receptor to cerebral cortex. DRG, dorsal root ganglion cells; IG, intermediate grey of the spinal cord; VHC, ventral horn motor neurons; VPL, ventroposterolateral nucleus of thalamus.

Another area of importance in sensory perception is the superior parietal lobule (area 5, 7).

c. The organization of fibers in the medial lemniscus which arises from cells of the nuclei cuneatus and gracilis and projects to the thalamus also shows a somatotopic localization as do the cells in the two nuclei.

d. The distribution of the neurons and fibers which transmit the sensations mediated through the dorsal column is illustrated in Figs 89—96.

e. Note in Figs 89—96 that the distribution of neurons and fibers that mediate unconscious position are also illustrated. In this instance collaterals of the fibers transmitting conscious proprioception or specific fibers terminate on cells of the nucleus dorsalis (of Clarke) at the base of the dorsal horn which then gives rise to projecting fibers which ascend ipsilaterally in the dorsal spinocerebellar tract. The nucleus dorsalis extends from the 1st thoracic to the 3rd lumbar segment of the spinal cord. There are further connections made on cells in the intermediate grey which send their axons contralaterally to ascend in the ventral spinocerebellar tract. Both of these

133

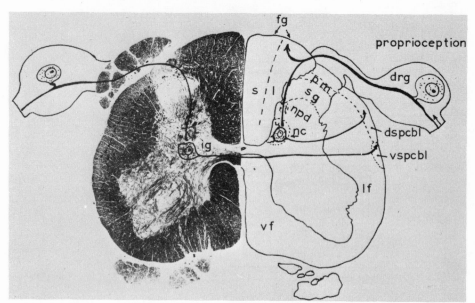

Fig. 89

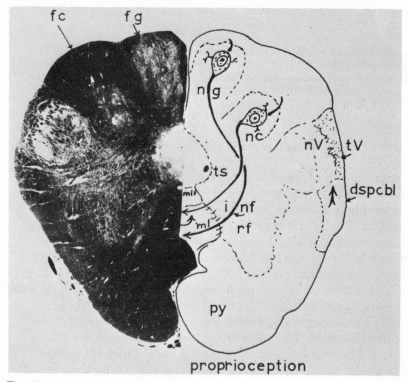

Fig. 90

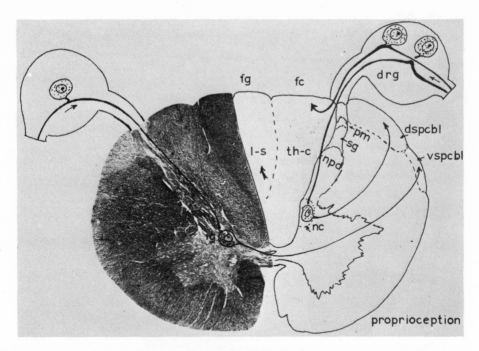

Fig. 91. An illustration of the cells and fiber tracts concerned with transmission of fine discriminative senses (+ unconscious proprioception) at the 1st or 2nd thoracic spinal cord level. Again a connection is illustrated for unconscious proprioception with a synapse occurring on cells in either the nucleus dorsalis or the intermediate grey. drg, dorsal root ganglion cell; dspcbl, dorsal spinocerebellar tract; fc, fasciculus cuneatus; fg, fasciculus gracilis; ig, intermediate grey; l-s, lumbosacral fibers; nc, nucleus dorsalis (of Clarke); npd, nucleus proprius dorsalis; pm, nucleus posteromarginalis; sg, substantia gelatinosa; th-c, thoracic and cervical fibers; vspcbl, ventral spinocerebellar tract.

Fig. 89. An illustration of the cells and fiber tracts concerned with transmission of fine discriminative senses (+ unconscious proprioception) at the 1st or 2nd lumbar spinal cord level. A collateral is shown coming off the primary dorsal column fiber tract to synapse on cells of the nucleus dorsalis (of Clarke) for transmission of unconscious proprioceptive sense to the cerebellum. drg, dorsal root ganglion cells; dspcbl, dorsal spinocerebellar tract; fg, fasciculus gracilis; ig, intermediate grey; l, lumbar fibers; lf, lateral funiculus; nc, nucleus dorsalis (of Clarke); npd, nucleus proprius dorsalis; pm, nucleus postero-marginalis; s, sacral fibers; sg, substantia gelatinosa; vf, ventral funiculus; vspcbl, ventro-spinal cerebellar tract.

Fig. 90. An illustration of the cells and fibers concerned with the transmission of discriminative sensation from the body at the level of the caudal closed medulla. dspcbl, dorsal spinocerebellar tract; fc, fasciculus cuneatus; fg, fasciculus gracilis; inf, internal arcuate nerve fibers; ml, medial lemniscus; mlf, medial longitudinal fasciculus; nc, nucleus cuneatus; ng, nucleus gracilis; nV, nucleus of the descending tract of the trigeminal nerve; py, pyramid; rf, reticular formation; ts, solitary tract and nucleus; tV, descending tract and nucleus of the trigeminal nerve.

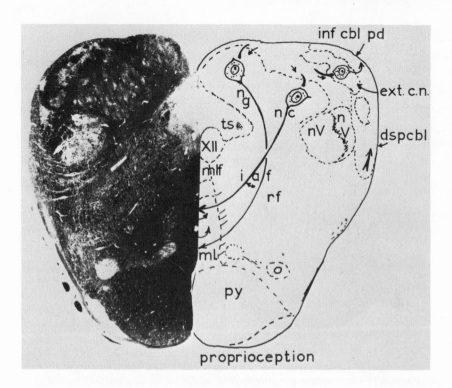

Fig. 92. An illustration of the cells and fibers concerned with the transmission of discriminative sensations from the body at the level of the closed medulla. Note connections coming in from the fasciculus cuneatus to terminate on cells of the external cuneate nucleus (ext. c.n.) which relay unconscious proprioceptive sensations from the neck regions to the cerebellum. dspcbl, dorsal spinocerebellar tract; iaf, internal arcuate nerve fibers; inf cbl pd, inferior cerebellar peduncle; ml, medial lemniscus; mlf, medial longitudinal fasciculus; nc, nucleus cuneatus; ng, nucleus gracilis; nV, nucleus of the descending tract of the trigeminal nerve; o, inferior olivary nucleus; py, pyramid; rf, reticular formation; ts, solitary tract and nucleus; tV, descending tract of the trigeminal nerve; XII, hypoglossal nerve nucleus.

tracts enter primarily into the inferior cerebellar peduncle (restiform body) to be distributed to the cerebellar cortex. A small proportion of the fibers in the ventral tract by-pass the inferior and middle cerebellar peduncles to enter the cerebellum via the superior peduncle (brachium conjunctivum).

(i) Note that fibers conveying unconscious proprioception from spinal cord segments L_4 to S_5 ascend in the dorsal funiculus to terminate in the nucleus dorsalis at the 3rd lumbar level inasmuch as the nucleus dorsalis is not present caudally. Further, comparable information entering the cord in the cervical cord also ascends in the dorsal funiculus without synapsing (again because the nucleus dorsalis is absent) to

136

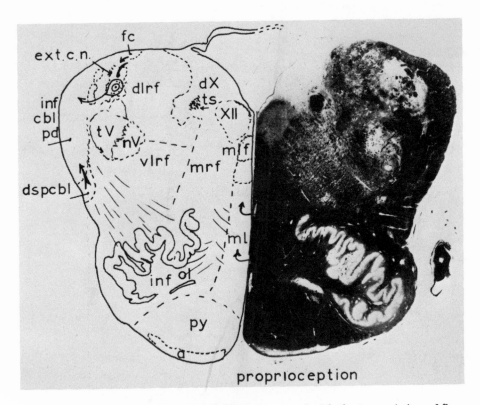

proprioception

Fig. 93. An illustration of the cells and fibers concerned with the transmission of fine discriminative sensations from the body at the level of the open medulla. Note fibers coming in from the fasciculus cuneatus (fc) to terminate on cells of the external cuneate nucleus (ext. c.n.) which relay unconscious proprioceptive sense to the cerebellum. a, arcuate nucleus; dlrf, dorsolateral reticular formation; dspcbl, dorsal spinocerebellar tract; dX, dorsal motor nucleus of the vagus nerve; inf cbl pd, inferior cerebellar peduncle; inf ol, inferior olivary nucleus; ml, medial lemniscus; mlf, medial longitudinal fasciculus; mrf, medial reticular formation; nV, nucleus of the descending tract of the trigeminal nerve; py, pyramid; ts, solitary tract and nucleus; tV, descending tract of the trigeminal nerve; XII, hypoglossal nerve nucleus.

terminate on cells of the external cuneate nucleus whose fibers then project into the inferior cerebellar peduncle.

(ii) Recent investigations on the pathways for tactile information which have classically been considered to pass primarily through the dorsal column have been shown in cat and dog and now in monkey to have an additional route (Andersson, 1972). On the basis of electrical physiological information there appears to be an input via the dorsal root which ascends ipsilaterally in the dorsal aspect of the lateral funiculus to the lateral cervical nucleus from which secondary fibers emerge and enter the medial lemniscus and thus reach the thalamus. A

137

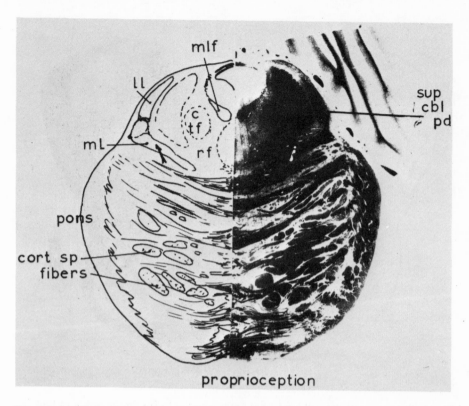

Fig. 94. An illustration of the cells and nerve fibers concerned with the transmission of discriminative sensations from the body at the level of the rostral pons. cort sp fibers, cortical spinal fibers; ctf, central tegmental fasciculus; LL, lateral lemniscus; mL, medial lemniscus; mlf, medial longitudinal fasciculus; rf, reticular formation; sup cbl pd, superior cerebellar peduncle.

second contralateral pathway has also been described which ascends in the ventral aspect of the lateral funiculus and has been shown to reach the sensory cortex. However, whatever way-stations for relay are in this path remain uncertain. These two alternative pathways are indicated in Fig. 88, but not in the subsequent Pal-Weigert projections. Perhaps these observations may explain the experience of neurosurgeons who have observed maintainance of dorsal column sensations after damage to the dorsal column.

C. Discriminative sensations arising from the face are also relayed to the cortex in a somatotopic manner via a tract system which is essentially crossed (Fig. 97). Note that unconscious position sense (proprioception) appears related to the cells of the mesencephalic nucleus which then effect reflex

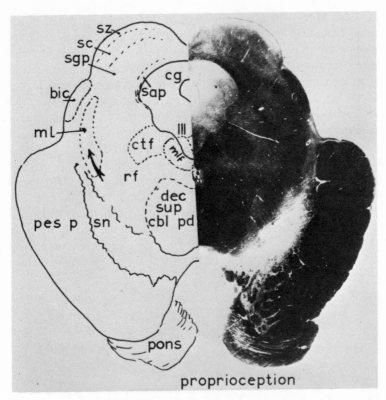

Fig. 95. An illustration of the cells and nerve fibers concerned with the transmission of discriminative sensations from the body at the level of the superior colliculus. bic, brachium of the inferior colliculus; cg, central grey; ctf, central tegmental fasciculus; dec sup cbl pd, decussation of the superior cerebellar peduncle; mL, medial lemniscus; mlf, medial longitudinal fasciculus; pes p, pes pedunculi; sap, stratum album profundum; sc, superior colliculus; sgp, stratum griseum profundum; sn, substantia nigra; sz, stratum zonale; III, oculomotor nucleus.

connections with the motor trigeminal nucleus and with other cranial nerve nuclei. Connections to the cerebellum also seem to be established, but by uncertain pathways. Conscious proprioceptive information would appear to reach the cortex in conjunction with the other discriminative sensations. While many sources describe the trigeminal projections as ascending via the dorsocentral trigeminal tract, the precise location of this tract in the brain stem remains ill-defined.

D. Visceral sensations. While our understanding of the distribution of afferents from visceral structures is far from complete, it is apparent that such afferents exist. By and large they are located in the splanchnic sympathetic nerves with cell bodies in the dorsal root ganglia. Afferents from the sigmoid, colon, rectum, neck of the bladder, prostate and cervix of the uterus enter the cord via the dorsal roots of the 2nd to the 4th sacral segments and peripherally are associated with the pelvic parasympathetic neurons rather than the sympathetic fibers. The vagus nerve provides one significant route for afferent input from the viscera, being of particular importance in cardiac and respiratory control. Afferents for taste enter the CNS via VII and IX, while IX also transmits afferents from the carotid sinus. Both VII and IX are involved with visceral afferents from mucous membranes of the mouth and pharyngeal wall. It is clear that some visceral afferent impulses are transmitted to higher levels of the CNS and ultimately attain the conscious level. However, the route whereby this occurs is uncertain. The general sensations transmitted are diffuse and relate to feelings of hunger, thirst, fullness of bladder and bowels, etc. In general, it would appear that the viscera are insensitive to touch or temperature and thus may be operated on under a local anesthesia without producing pain, unless the parietal, peritoneal, pleural or pericardial membranes are manipulated. However, violent pain is known to be associated with visceral organs.

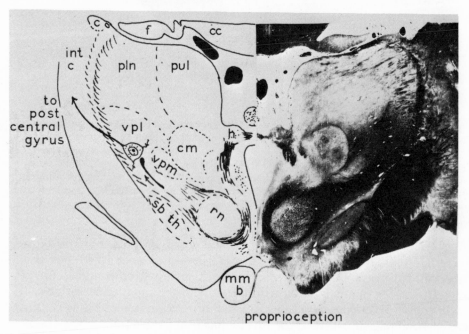

Fig. 96. An illustration of the cells and fibers concerned with the transmission of discriminative senses from the body to the cortex at the level of the caudal thalamus. c, caudate nucleus; cc, corpus callosum; cm, centromedial nucleus of thalamus (centrum medianum); f, fornix; h, habenular nucleus of epithalamus; int c, internal capsule; mmb, mammillary bodies; pln, posterolateral nucleus of thalamus; pul, pulvinar of thalamus; rn, red nucleus; sb th, subthalamic nucleus; vpl, ventroposterolateral nucleus of thalamus; vpm, ventroposteromedial nucleus of thalamus.

140

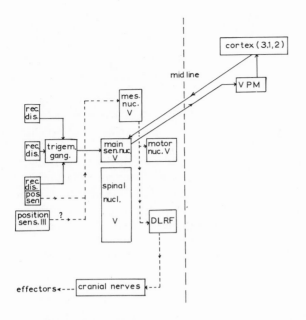

Fig. 97. A schematic illustration of the major components concerned with the transmission of discriminative sensations from the face. DLRF, dorsolateral reticular formation; main sen. nuc. V, main trigeminal sensory nucleus; mes. nuc. V, mesencephalic trigeminal sensory nucleus; pos sen, position sense; rec dis., receptor for discriminative senses; spinal nucl. V, descending spinal trigeminal sensory nucleus; trigem. gang., trigeminal ganglion; VPM, ventroposteromedial nucleus of thalamus.

This seems to be related to distension of the hollow visceral structures which may set up forcible contractions of the smooth muscles in the walls (spasms), pinching nerve endings. The rapid stretching of the capsules to such organs as the spleen and liver similarly may produce pain. Anoxemia of the heart muscle is also associated with severe pain. While visceral pain is frequently diffusely localized by the patient, there is often an irradiation of the pain to a cutaneous area. This pain is termed referred pain.

1. Some common sites of referred pain are as follows.
    a. Medial aspect of the left arm and left chest from cardiac anoxemia (angina pectoris).
    b. Pain in the right scapular region for disease of the liver or gall bladder.
    c. Epigastric pain with gastric ulcers or other gastric disease.
    d. Inguinal or testicular pain in renal colic.
    e. Pain at the base of the neck with inflammation or disease affecting the diaphragm.
    f. Pain in the lower right abdominal quadrant with appendicitis.

141

2. Explanations for referred pain have yet to delineate the cause clearly. However, there may be some relation to the site of somatic pain induced by the visceral disturbance to a common spinal cord level of innervation. Thus, as cited by Head, the painful cutaneous areas or zones associated with pain from the various visceral organs coincide roughly with the segmental distribution of the somatic sensory fibers which arise from the cord at the same level as the fibers of the splanchnic nerves which go to the viscera. Further, as suggested by Mackenzie, abnormally strong visceral input arising from a diseased visceral organ may produce some increased irritability (decreased threshold) in the neurons of the dorsal horn such that subliminal stimuli from the cutaneous structures innervated by neurons terminating at the same segmental level may be perceived and interpreted as painful. Another suggestion which has been made is that the visceral input may induce reflex spasmodic contractions of muscles underlying the cutaneous referred pain area which then leads to excessive stimulation of pain receptors in the involved muscles and to real pain.

E. Clinical correlations of somatic afferent systems.

1. Irritative lesions of the dorsal roots from compression, traction, inflammation or by interference in blood supply lead to radicular pain related to the specific roots involved. This may be observed in the early stages of tabes dorsalis (syphilis of the CNS) when the involvement is still restricted to the meninges. However, with tabes there is eventually a complete loss of sensation as the roots and dorsal root ganglia become destroyed.

a. Irritation of the dorsal root does not necessarily lead to pain but may cause paresthesia: a feeling of numbness, pricking, tingling, etc.

b. Since the fibers of a single dorsal root segment overlap the next root segments caudally and rostrally, the loss of a single root would not lead to an absolute loss of sensation, though there may be a limited zone of changes in sensation.

c. Compression, vascular or degenerative lesions may also affect the fibers of the ascending anterolateral fasciculus and thus produce a contralateral loss of pain and temperature below the level of the lesion. Similar lesions may occur on either side of the dorsal funiculus to produce an ipsilateral loss of discriminatory sensations below the level of the lesion. Comparable situations may also occur in the medial lemniscus at any level to produce contralateral losses of discriminatory sensations.

(i) Vascular lesions frequently occur in the dorsolateral quadrant of the medulla as a result of a pathologic state of the posterior inferior cerebellar artery. Such encephalomalacic areas of focal degeneration produce ipsilateral loss of pain and temperature from the face, a contralateral loss of pain and temperature from the body, plus vestibular, auditory and cerebellar symptoms due to the close proximity of tracts from these systems in the same region.

(ii) Vascular disease leading to encephalomalacic degeneration may also occur in the specific relay nuclei of the thalamus, in the internal capsule or in the primary sensory cortex.

2. Lesions of the central grey of the spinal cord. These are frequently associated with syringomyelia in which there is a cavitation of the spinal cord around the central canal which intersects the secondary decussating fibers transmitting pain and temperature. Thus, there is a segmental loss of pain and temperature extending throughout the entire course of the lesion. The cavitation is progressive and thus may eventually affect the motor cells of the ventral horn (lower motor neuron paralysis) or the descending cortico-spinal fibers of the lateral funiculus (upper motor neuron paralysis). Such cavitations may also occur in the medulla.

3. Alcoholic neuropathy. Acute alcoholism influences both the sensory and motor nerves and seems clearly related to the nutritional deficiency of the B complex vitamins and partly to disturbances in glucose metabolism. The effect is most severe distally so that extensors of the feet and toes are most affected, with extensors of the wrist being next. Flexor muscles of the fingers are also often involved. Sensory input from the hands and feet is similarly most affected involving both position sense and pain and temperature. The sensory and motor losses are both associated with demyelinization. If the disease does not proceed too far, considerable recovery may be expected with vitamin B therapy and proper diet. However, in long protracted cases the neurons will also undergo degeneration.

a. Both the myelin sheath and the axon are involved in alcoholic neuropathy though the axonal changes appear later. The fact that the axon also undergoes degeneration may explain why vitamin B therapy has little effect except during the early stages of the disease.

b. Alcohol is also toxic to neurons and is known to suppress protein and RNA synthesis which, if continued, must eventually disrupt the biochemical and physiological integrity of neurons.

Chapter 12

THE VISUAL PATHWAYS

A. The eyeball.

 1. Gross structure. The eye is a highly developed mobile receptor adapted for detection of distant stimuli, an exteroceptor. The gross structural components are illustrated in Fig. 98. It should be noted that the eye has three separate refractive media.

 a. The cornea at the anterior pole with a refractive index of 1.376 as compared to an index of 1.0 for air. The cornea is the most important refractive element of the eye.

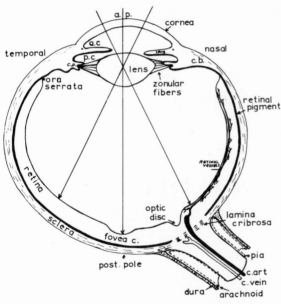

Fig. 98. A diagrammatic illustration of a cross-section through the eyeball showing the principal gross elements. Note that the passage of light rays through the refractive media of the cornea, lens and vitreous humor reverses the image which impinges upon the retina. Also note that the dura of the CNS fuses to the sclera at the exit of the optic nerve and that the other CNS meningeal membranes are present around the optic nerve, thus providing for a subarachnoid space around the nerve. Note further that the region of greatest visual acuity in the retina occurs at the fovea centralis and that there are no visual receptor elements at the optic disc. a.c., anterior chamber; a.p., anterior pole; c.b., ciliary body; c.p., ciliary processes; fovea c., fovea centralis; p.c., posterior chamber; c. art, central retinal artery; c. vein, central retinal vein.

145

b. The crystalline lens with a refractive index of 1.36 in the peripheral layers and of 1.4 in the inner zone is the second most important refractive element of the eye.

c. The vitreous body which fills the cavity between the lens and the retina is the third refractive element of the eye with a refractive index of 1.334.

d. The anterior and the posterior chambers of the eye are filled with the transparent aqueous humor.

e. Note that the outer surface of the retina is pigmented and that the retina is finally ensheathed in a tough connective capsule (sclera) which forms the outer layer of the eyeball. The anterior margin of the sclera is modified to form the cornea. Posteriorly it is perforated at the lamina cribrosa by nerve fibers arising from ganglion cells.

2. The retina, which is virtually transparent in life except for the outer pigmented zone, contains the cells which are the receptor elements. The area

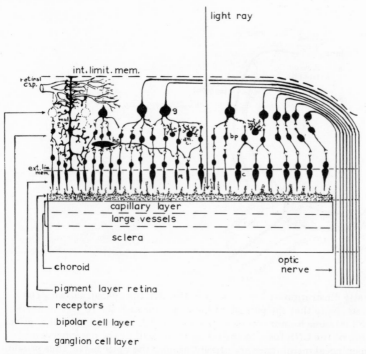

Fig. 99. A schematic diagram of the retina. Note that the light rays pass through the entire retina before they can stimulate the rod (R) or cone (C) cells. am. c., amacrine cell; bp, bipolar neuron; ext. lim. mem., external limiting membrane; g, ganglion neuron of retina; hc, horizontal cell; int. limit. mem., internal limiting membrane; mül. f., Müller fiber (glial cell).

146

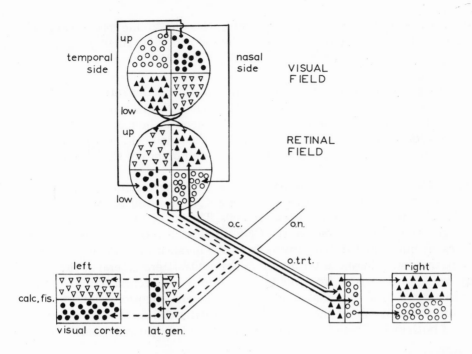

Fig. 100. A schematic diagram illustrating the reversal of image from the visual field to the retinal field. Note that in the subsequent projection the nasal fibers cross and the temporal retinal fibers remain ipsilateral. calc. fis., calcarine fissure and adjacent visual cortex; lat. gen., lateral geniculate body; o.c., optic chiasm; o.n., optic nerve; o. trt., optic tract.

of greatest visual acuity (where receptors for color vision have a one to one to one relationship between cone cells, bipolar neurons and ganglion cells) is at the fovea centralis. The anterior margin of the retina at the ora serrata is the region where visual acuity is least. It is, however, most sensitive to stimuli in light of low intensity. Note that the various refractive media (cornea, lens and vitreous body) invert the image as they project it toward the retinal surface (Figs 98 and 100) so that the left side of the visual field impinges on the right retinal field and that the upper visual field stimulates cells of the lower retinal field. Thus, the temporal side of the visual field projects onto the nasal retina, etc.

 a. The organization of the retina is schematically portrayed by Fig. 99. Note that the part of the retina near the exit of the projection fibers arising from ganglion cells has a higher concentration of cone receptor cells which have a one to one relationship with bipolar cells. The bipolar cells then have a one to one relationship with ganglion cells. This would be most evident in the macula lutea of the fovea centralis.

147

More peripherally (toward the ora serrata) this one to one relationship is lost and the primary receptor element is the rod cell. Note further that the light rays must pass through the entire retina before they are in a position to stimulate the receptor cells.

(i) The vascular supply to the retina from the retinal artery is more or less limited to the layer of large ganglion cells. Nourishment of the bipolar neurons, rod and cone cells then seems to be mediated by transport through the Müller fibers (modified glial cells) which also give rise to the internal and external limiting membranes of the retina.

B. The pathway. Light stimuli entering the eye impinge on the retina to activate cone and rod receptor cells, which in turn transmit the stimuli to the bipolar cells and thence to the ganglion cells. The latter are the large cells which give rise to a large tract of the CNS, the so-called optic nerve, which is not a nerve but a tract. Fibers arising from the nasal surfaces of the retina cross in the optic chiasm to terminate in the contralateral lateral geniculate body, while fibers arising from the temporal side of the retina terminate in the ipsilateral lateral geniculate body. By this means, the projection of an object in the right side of the visual field stimulates cells in the left retinal field, of both eyes. These fields (temporal for the left eye and nasal for the

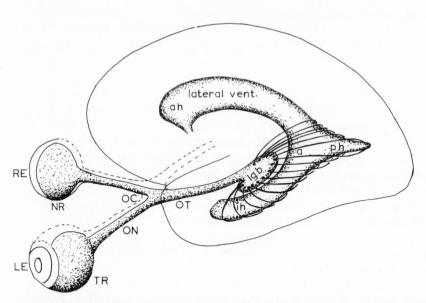

Fig. 101. A diagrammatic representation of the course of the optic radiations in relation to the lateral ventricle. a, antrum; ah, anterior horn of lateral ventricle; ih, inferior horn of lateral ventricle; LE, left eye; lgb, lateral geniculate body; NR, nasal retina; OC, optic chiasm; ON, optic nerve; OT, optic tract; ph, posterior horn of lateral ventricle; RE, right eye; TR, temporal retina.

148

right eye) then relay the information via the left optic tract to left lateral geniculate body and then through the left optic radiation to the left visual cortex surrounding the calcarine fissure of the occipital lobe.

1. The course of the optic radiations through the brain occupies an extensive area (Fig. 101). Thus, fibers from the lateral side of the geniculate body course down into the temporal lobe, passing over the inferior horn of the lateral ventricle and then course caudally to pass under the posterior horn of the lateral ventricle to reach the medial occipital temporal gyrus (lingual gyrus). Fibers from the medial aspect of the geniculate body pass laterally around the antrum of the lateral ventricle and then turn caudally to pass over the dorsal aspect of the posterior horn of the lateral ventricle to terminate in the cuneus. This wide divergence of fibers in the temporal, parietal and occipital lobes makes the visual pathway subject to damage from lesions of the CNS at a number of points. Thus, visual symptoms commonly occur from lesions in either the temporal, parietal or occipital lobes.

a. Rule of L. When referring to the projections of the retina to the visual cortex, it is sometimes handy to remember this mnemonic: Lower retinal fibers project to the Lateral part of the lateral geniculate body, which relays them through the Lower part of the optic radiations through the temporal lobe to the Lingual gyrus which is the lowermost part of the visual cortex. However, since the lens system reverses the image as it projects onto the retina, this lower retinal projection relates to the upper visual field. The upper retinal projection must then logically relate to the rest of the pathway and to the lower visual field.

C. Some of the various types of visual defects which may be encountered are summarized in Fig. 102. These range from scotomata wherein there is an area of damaged retina leading to a blind (dark) spot in a particular eye to an anopsia (*an* non-use + *opsia* sight) of one eye or a hemi- (half) anopsia in a particular visual field. If the field loss is the same in both eyes it is termed homonymous (meaning same), while if the field loss is different in the two eyes (i.e. left visual field in the left eye and right visual field in the right eye which would be bitemporal) the term applied is heteronymous, meaning different for the two eyes in relation to the side of the visual field lost.

1. A damaged portion of the retina producing a scotoma. Could be due to a mechanical or vascular lesion.

2. Severance of the optic nerve leading to an anopsia of that eye. Again, this could be due to a mechanical injury, either to the nerve or to the eyeball.

3. Severance of the fibers crossing in the optic chiasm as might occur with a pituitary tumor leading to a bitemporal heteronymous hemianopsia.

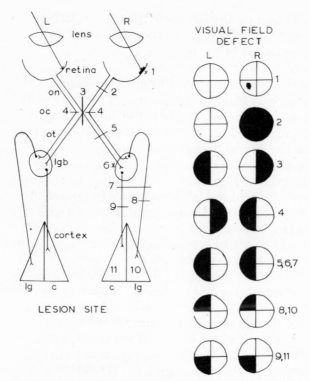

Fig. 102. A schematic outline of the visual system illustrating the visual field defects occurring with various lesions of the system. c, cuneus; L, left; lg, lingual gyrus (medial occipital temporal gyrus); lgb, lateral geniculate body; oc, optic chiasm; on, optic nerve; ot, optic tract; R, right. Lesions: 1, localized damage to retina producing a scotoma; 2, severance of optic nerve producing an ipsilateral blindness; 3, pressure on the medial aspect of the chiasm producing a bitemporal heteronymous hemianopsia (possibly by a pituitary tumor); 4, pressure on the chiasm (possibly from two aneurysms of the internal carotid arteries) producing a binasal heteronymous hemianopsia; 5, severance of the optic tract (right) producing a left homonymous hemianopsia; 6, damage to the right lateral geniculate body and 7, damage to the right optic radiations would have the same effect as the damage to the tract at 5; 8, damage to the lower optic radiations or damage to the lingual gyrus (10) would both produce an upper left homonymous quadranopsia; 9, damage to the upper half of the optic radiations or to the cuneus (11) would both produce a lower left homonymous quadranopsia when the damage occurs on the right side, as illustrated.

4. Severance of the uncrossed fibers at the optic chiasm as might occur with bilateral aneurysms of the internal carotid arteries to produce a binasal heteronymous hemianopsia.

5. Severance of the right optic tract to produce a left homonymous hemianopsia. This could be caused by pressure from a tumor lodged within the temporal lobe against the optic tract.

150

6. Damage to the right lateral geniculate body resulting from vascular insufficiency or the presence of some other form of lesion to cause a left homonymous hemianopsia.

7. Damage to the entire right optic radiation from intracerebral hemorrhage to produce a left homonymous hemianopsia.

8. Damage to the right lower optic radiation in the temporal lobe due to vascular or tumour etiology (etc.) to produce a left upper homonymous quadranopsia (quarter field loss).

9. Damage to the right upper component of the optic radiation caused by the presence of some lesion in the right parietal and adjacent occipital lobe to produce a left lower homonymous quadranopsia.

10. Damage at the level of the right visual cortex in the lingual gyrus (medial occipital temporal gyrus) to produce an upper left homonymous quadranopsia.

11. Damage to the right cuneus to produce a lower left homonymous quadranopsia.
    a. Both the latter two lesions may be encountered with thrombosis of a branch of the posterior cerebral artery. However, it is more common to find that the entire visual cortex on the affected side is infarcted, thus producing a hemianopsia. Small meningiomas in the falx cerebri or leptomeninges have also been observed to have localized effects on vision at the level of the primary visual cortex (area 17). Such lesions impinging on the secondary visual cortex (area 18 or 19) have been reported to cause difficulties in visual perception without blindness.

12. Edema of the optic disc. The axons of retinal ganglion cells form a small disc at the site of exit from the retina. This may become swollen if there is an increase in intracerebral pressure. Such an increase in pressure in the CSF will cause a compression of the optic nerves because they are encased with meninges and possess a subarachnoid space. The resulting increase in CSF pressure compresses the central retinal vein more than the artery, thus allowing more blood to enter the retina than leaves it. This disturbance in hemodynamics causes edema manifested by swelling of the optic disc (choked disc).

D. Reflex connections.

1. The light reflex consists of the reflex constriction of the pupil when a bright light is shone upon it. The response which occurs in the eye upon which

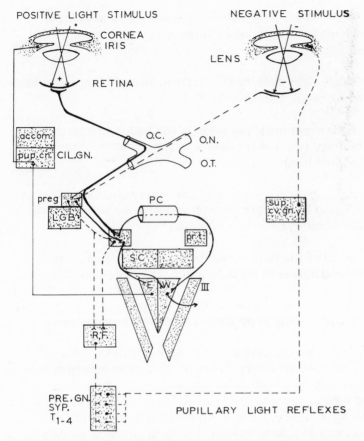

POSITIVE LIGHT STIMULUS NEGATIVE STIMULUS

CORNEA
IRIS
LENS
RETINA

accom.
pup.cn. CIL.GN.
O.C.
O.N.
O.T.

preg
LGB
PC
prt.
sup.
cv.gn.
SC
E W III
R.F.

PRE.GN.
SYP.
T_{1-4} PUPILLARY LIGHT REFLEXES

Fig. 103. A diagrammatic representation of the CNS connections concerned with the pupillary light reflex. The figure includes a potential sympathetic relay series which might be invoked under circumstances where light intensity is very low. accom., portion of the ciliary ganglion containing cells involved in accommodation; CIL.GN., ciliary ganglion; EW, nucleus of Edinger and Westphal; LGB, lateral geniculate body; PC, posterior commissure; preg, pregeniculate nucleus; PRE.GN.SYP., preganglionic sympathetic neurons; prt, pretectal area; pup. cn., cells of ciliary ganglion associated with pupillary constriction; R.F., reticular formation; sup. cv. gn., superior cervical ganglion; III, oculomotor nucleus.

the light is directed is the direct reflex. A comparable response may be observed in the unstimulated eye. This is the consensual reflex and is presumed to occur because of connections from the pretectal area on the stimulated side through the posterior commissure to the contralateral pretectal area. One should also note, however, that the pretectal area probably innervates the parasympathetic preganglionic nucleus of Edinger and Westphal bilaterally. Note in Fig. 103 that the input from the retina which induces this reflex response by-passes the lateral geniculate body to terminate directly in the

152

pretectal area. (Some connections in a pregeniculate nucleus have been described by some authors which serve to relay a part of this type of information to the pretectal area. This would seem to be a minor contribution to the reflex pathway.) Note that the efferent fibers from the nucleus of Edinger and Westphal relay the signal through a part of the ciliary ganglion, which has been reported by Warwick to contain specific cells for the light reflex and other cells for the accommodation reflex.

a. The effect of an absence of light. This produces a pupillary dilation and for many years has been assumed to be related to direct innervation of

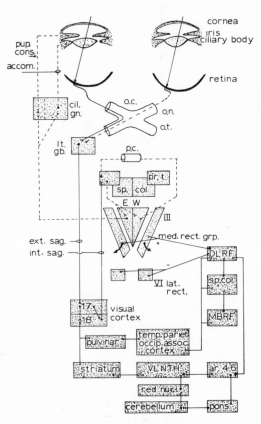

Fig. 104. A diagrammatic representation of the CNS connections concerned with the accommodation reflex. accom., fibers going from cells of ciliary ganglion associated with changes in lens thickness; cil. gn., ciliary ganglion; DLRF, dorsolateral reticular formation; ext. sag., external sagittal stratum of optic radiation; EW, nucleus of Edinger and Westphal; int. sag., internal sagittal stratum of optic radiation; lt. gb., lateral geniculate body; med. rect. grp., medial rectus associated cells of oculomotor nucleus; MBRF, midbrain reticular formation; o.c., optic chiasm; o.n., optic nerve; o.t., optic tract; p.c., posterior commissure; pr. t., pretectal area; sp. col., superior colliculus; III, oculomotor nucleus; VI lat. rect., abducens nucleus innervation of lateral rectus muscle.

153

dilator muscles mediated through the sympathetic system from preganglionics found in the intermediolateral cell column in the first four thoracic segments of the spinal cord (Fig. 103). These then are presumed to act via postganglionic neurons in the superior cervical ganglion. Recent studies suggest, however, that the effect of the dilator muscle is probably minimal and that pupillary constriction and dilation may be primarily due to tonic regulation of the parasympathetic constrictor component, since pupillary dilation is still possible after destruction of the superior cervical ganglion. Despite these observations it should be noted that active sympathetic stimulation will induce pupillary dilation. This response may be related to the sympathetic innervation of the blood vessels supplying the ciliary ganglion. Thus, a reduction of blood supply to the ganglion may be thought of as decreasing the activity of these postganglionic neurons which innervate the pupillary constrictor muscle, and so lead to pupillary dilation.

2. The accommodation reflex is the other major reflex mechanism of the eye. It involves pupillary constriction, adjustments of the lens and convergence of the eyes to bring both eyes to focus on the same object. The connections for these responses are schematically summarized in Fig. 104. Note that the reflex response, unlike the light reflex, requires a cortical connection through the optic radiation which provides for a relatively simple relay back to the pretectal area. Note that the fibers directed toward the cortex pass through that part of the optic radiation frequently referred to as the external sagittal stratum. The returning fibers from area 18 pass through what is often termed the internal sagittal stratum. In addition, there are connections to provide for some very complicated interactions to ensure proper organization of the activity of neurons innervating the extraocular muscles in a coordinated fashion. The indicated proposed connections for providing the appropriate response of nerves innervating the extraocular muscles are speculative, but based on known anatomical connections. However, it is not yet clear whether these pathways are utilized in the physiological response of convergence. Note further that both cell groups of the ciliary ganglion (those for pupillary constriction and those for change in lens shape) are involved in the reflex.

a. A center for convergence was believed to exist in the oculomotor nucleus for many years (nucleus of Perlia). However, investigations by Warwick have demonstrated that the connections of this nucleus could not provide for convergence. Thus, it would appear that the convergence portion of the reflex is not controlled at a midbrain level, but probably at a higher level such as visual cortex, thalamus or striatum.

3. Clinical associations. Various components of these reflex responses may be interfered with by small lesions of a vascular or tumorous nature though this should not be considered to be an exclusive etiology. Such lesions may literally occur at any site in the pathway and may interfere to a greater or

154

lesser degree with the response. However, the midbrain is the most common site.

a. The Argyll Robertson pupil is a condition which occurs in tertiary syphilis (syphilis of the nervous system) in which the pupil is small and irregularly constricted and fails to respond to light, but is said to respond in accommodation, thus suggesting that the pathway for the constriction which occurs in accommodation is different from that which occurs with the light reflex. The significance of this observation is perhaps open to some question, since the Argyll Robertson pupil is virtually maximally constricted and could hardly be expected to constrict further just because the type of stimulus applied is different. What seems to be suggested is that the tonic control mediated by the parasympathetic neurons is no longer functioning in the appropriate manner and thus fails to allow for a relaxation of the pupillary constrictor muscles.

b. The Adie pupil may be mistaken for the Argyll Robertson pupil as it too shows a disturbance in the reaction to light and shows a preservation of the accommodation reflex. However, the Adie pupil will dilate slowly in a dark room and then constrict slowly in response to a bright light.

Chapter 13

THE AUDITORY PATHWAYS

The detection of sound depends on the translation of sound waves in the air, which are picked up by the external ear (ExE in Fig. 105), to a mechanical wave by the bony ossicles (malleus, m; incus, in; stapes, s) of the middle ear (ME). This mechanical energy is then relayed by vibration of the stapes against the membrane covering the oval window which in turn elicts comparable vibrations in the perilymph of the scala vestibuli (sv) and scala tympani of the inner ear (InE). These vibrations in turn induce vibrations in the basilar membrane (bm) on which rests the sensory receptor for hearing, the Organ of Corti (or cor). Hairs arising from hair cells in the Organ of Corti are embedded in the tectorial membrane (tm₂). The movement of the basilar membrane is greater along its lateral than its medial edge which is attached to a bony lamina. Thus, the movements of the hair cells and their hairs in relation to the

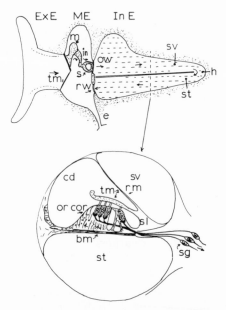

Fig. 105. A diagrammatic representation of the anatomical components of the ear and the Organ of Corti. bm, basilar membrane; cd, cochlear duct; e, eustachian tube; ExE, external ear; h, helicotrema; in, incus; InE, inner ear; m, malleus; ME, middle ear; or cor, Organ of Corti; ow, oval window; rw, round window; sg, spiral ganglion; sl, limbus laminae spiralis; st, scala tympani; sv, scala vestibuli; tm₁, tympanic membrane; tm₂, tectorial membrane.

157

tectorial membrane are such that there is a lateral shearing movement as well as an up and down movement. In some way this activates the neuronal terminals at the bases of the hair cells to transmit a signal toward the CNS relative to the quality and intensity of the sound. The cell bodies for these neurons are located in a spiral bony cavity in the modiolus, forming the spiral ganglion (sg). The modiolus itself forms a type of hub around which the coils of the cochlear duct are wrapped.

A. Organization of the Organ of Corti

1. The sensory receptor organ sits on the basilar membrane, which is somewhat triangular in shape, increasing in width from its base near the oval window to its apex at the helicotrema. The receptor cells which are held by supporting cells on the basilar membrane are arranged in such a manner that those nearest the oval window respond to higher tones and finally to lower tones as the broader part of the membrane is reached at its apex. Thus, there is a tonotopic localization of receptors within the Organ of Corti.

2. Most of the dendritic endings of the ganglion cells are distributed to only a few hair cells in small groups. These fibers tend to run out radially from the ganglion cells to terminate on those hair cells closest to them. Other ganglion cells send their dendrites for some distance, along the cochlear duct and terminate on a number of cells spanning several tonotopic zones.

3. There are about 25 000 hair cells and 32 000 ganglion cells and fibers in man.

B. Central pathways. The connections from the cochlear nuclei in the medulla to higher centers are illustrated in Fig. 106.

1. The tonotopic distribution for sound observation in the receptors is maintained in the cochlear nucleus and in the auditory cortex (transverse temporal gyrus of Heschl, areas 41 and 42).

2. Note the multiple connections and bilateral projections which occur in the brain stem. This makes it very difficult to produce deafness by central lesions, except at the cochlear nuclei where vascular lesions associated with primary disease of the basilar artery or tumors of the VIIIth nerve (acoustic neurinomas) may produce an ipsilateral deafness. Cortical lesions in areas 41 and 42 distort the quality of sound or may make it difficult to determine the source of a sound.

3. Stimulation of the cortex in the parietal or temporal lobe has been reported to elicit impulses in the superior olivary nucleus. This nucleus gives

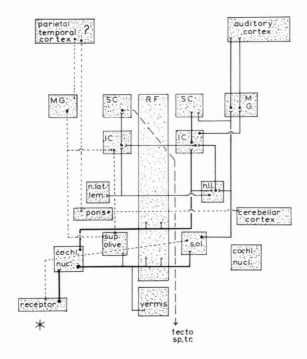

rise to the olivocochlear bundle which is primarily crossed, though there are some ipsilateral fibers. These efferent fibers terminate on the sensory hair cells in the Organ of Corti and have an inhibitory effect upon them.

4. Pathologic states. The auditory process may be disturbed by inflammation (infective) or degenerative processes involving the cochlea or the labyrinth, thus destroying or affecting the receptor organ. Further, there may be arthritic changes in the joints of the ear ossicles disturbing their normal function. In addition, the eardrum (tympanic membrane) may itself be damaged.

Chapter 14

INTEGRATION OF SENSORY INFORMATION

   The nature of the organization of the CNS is such that there is an extreme
degree of integration of the various levels of the CNS to each other as well as
of the different modalities of sensory or motor organization. To some extent
this is illustrated in Fig. 107 for the somatic, auditory and visual sensory
modalities. Somatic input is indicated as terminating in Brodmann areas 3,
1 and 2. This cortical region then establishes contact with areas 5 and 7,
which might be considered to be a psychic area. Visual input to area 17 is
likewise relayed to an adjacent psychic area, area 18. The same occurs with
auditory input which is relayed from area 41 to 42. These so-called psychic
areas then demonstrate a common type of connection in that they all
project to the pulvinar and posterolateral nucleus of the thalamus. From the
thalamus there are then established connections to the inferior parietal
lobules (associated with speech in the left hemisphere), to the frontal motor
and premotor areas and to area 22 of the temporal gyrus. Area 22 then
establishes connections with the dorsomedial nucleus of the thalamus which

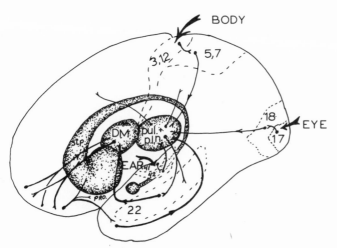

Fig. 107. A schematic illustration of the connections established from the primary cortices
for somatic sensation, vision and auditory sensations to secondary psychic cortical areas
which establish relays back to the diencephalon. This seems to serve as a means for
eventually relaying information to the frontal cortex and then into the motor system via
the basal nuclei and into the hypothalamus via the preoptic area. DM, dorsomedial nucleus
of thalamus; p.l.n., posterolateral nucleus of thalamus; pro., preoptic area; pul., pulvinar
of thalamus; stp., striatopallidum (basal ganglia). **Numbers refer to the Brodmann areas.**

is reciprocally connected with the frontal polar and orbital cortex. From the orbital cortex additional connections are made with the corpus striatum (striopallidum) and with the preoptic area, which is itself closely associated with hypothalamic function. Thus, the afferent input for somatic, visual and auditory sensations may influence or relate to the subsequent functions of the cortical areas concerned with language function, motor or higher activities, as well as with the functioning of the hypothalamus and autonomic system.

Chapter 15

THE VESTIBULAR CONNECTIONS

The vestibular component of the vestibulocochlear nerve (VIII) is better known for its reflex connections than for its projections to higher centers. However, there seems no doubt but that stimuli which activate the vestibular apparatus are appreciated at cortical levels. Impulses which arise from the vestibular apparatus of the inner ear come from two sorts of structure. One arises from stimulation of the crista of the ampullae of the semicircular canals. In this instance, hair cells of the receptors are stimulated by movements of the gelatinous cupula in which the hair processes are embedded. These are related to rotary movements of the head in any of three planes (angular acceleratory or deceleratory receptors). The other type of receptors, the maculae, are in sac-like dilations (the saccule and utricle) of the membranous labyrinth. The hair cells of these receptors also penetrate into a gelatinous mass, which contains many crystals of calcium carbonate (otoliths). These receptors are stimulated by nonrotatory movements of the head, up, down or sideways (position receptors). Terminal connections of bipolar neurons are established around the hair cells. The cell bodies of the neurons are located in the ganglion of Scarpa (vestibular ganglion).

A. The afferent pathway. The central processes of the bipolar cells terminate on cells of the flocculus and nodulus, on cells of the fastigial nucleus or on cells which form the four vestibular nuclei of the brain stem (Fig. 108). These are the superior, medial, lateral and inferior (descending) nuclei (schematized as a single nucleus in Fig. 108). While all nuclei receive primary vestibular afferents, not all cells within the nuclei receive terminals from the VIIIth nerve. These nuclei then give rise to fibers which are directed medially to form bundles of fibers which ascend or descend in a parasagittal position closely related to cranial nerve motor nuclei or the ventral horn of the spinal cord. Vestibular input has been shown to reach all of the cranial nerve motor nuclei. This is via the medial longitudinal fasciculus, termed the medial vestibulospinal tract in the cord. The medial vestibulospinal tract descends only to the cervical level and seems to be primarily derived bilaterally from cells of the medial vestibular nucleus. The lateral vestibular nucleus (of Deiters) gives rise to the lateral vestibulospinal tract which extends to the lumbosacral level and is known to increase extensor tonus of the limbs ipsilaterally.

B. The efferent vestibular component. There are also efferent neurons within the vestibular nerve, which arises from three small cell groups (one in the

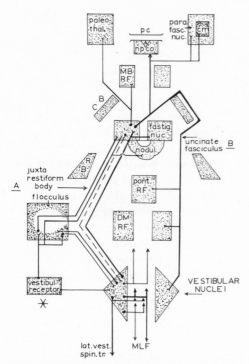

Fig. 108. A schematic illustration of the connections established within the CNS subsequent to vestibular stimulation. BC, brachium conjunctivum (superior cerebellar peduncle); CM, centrum medianum of thalamus (central medial nucleus); DMRF, dorso-medial reticular formation; lat. vest. spin. tr., lateral vestibulospinal tract; MBRF, midbrain reticular formation; MLF, medial longitudinal fasciculus; npco, nucleus of the posterior commissure; paleothal., paleothalamic nuclei of the internal and external medullary laminae; para. fasc. nuc., parafascicular nucleus; pont. RF, pontine reticular formation; RB, restiform body (inferior cerebellar peduncle).

lateral nucleus) to be distributed through the nerve to the vestibular sensory epithelium. Presumably these connections provide for some sort of central control over the receptor.

C. The various types of interconnections achieved by the vestibular system are illustrated by Fig. 108. This includes a somewhat ill-defined projection to the thalamus. While the pathways are uncertain, it also appears that perception of vestibular stimulation does reach the cortex, being almost exclusively contralateral in projection.

D. Reflex connections.

   1. One important reflex connection from the vestibular nuclei is to the nuclei giving rise to the nerves innervating the extraocular muscles.

Fig. 109 illustrates certain data from physiologic experiments and shows how connections from the ampullae of the various semicircular canals become associated with specific motor nerve nuclei to effect specific movements of the eye. In a later anatomical study (Fig. 110) it was demonstrated that all of the vestibular nuclei contribute to the ascending component of the medial longitudinal fasciculus and that all but the superior nucleus have bilateral projections. It can be appreciated from such anatomical connections how the vestibular complex is in a position to influence eye movements.

2. Another important series of reflex connections relates to the involvement of the vestibular system with motion sickness. Thus, reticular and vestibular neurons contribute an input via the medial longitudinal fasciculus to the motor nucleus of the trigeminal nerve (V), to the facial nerve (VII), to the

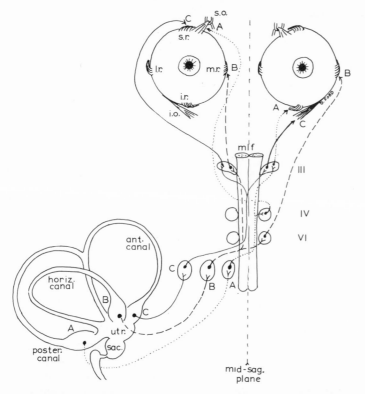

Fig. 109. A schematic illustration (based on Szentagothai) of a proposed interaction between the horizontal, anterior and posterior semicircular canals of the vestibular apparatus. A, B and C represent the vestibular nuclei in a general sense and only serve to indicate, for example, that canal A is related to some part of the vestibular nuclear complex which is then in turn related to those extraocular muscles indicated by A. i.o., inferior oblique muscle; i.r., inferior rectus muscle; l.r., lateral rectus muscle; mlf, medial longitudinal fasciculus; m.r., medial rectus muscle; sac., saccule; s.o., superior oblique muscle; s.r., superior rectus muscle; utr., utricle; III, oculomotor nucleus; IV, trochlear nucleus; VI, abducens nucleus.

165

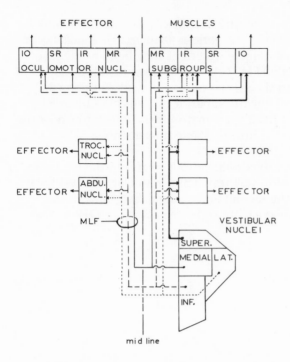

Fig. 110. A schematic illustration (based on McMasters *et al.*) of the connections between the various vestibular nuclei and the neurons innervating the different extraocular muscles. The quality of the line from a particular vestibular nucleus to a particular motor cell group has no relation to the number of fibers involved. ABDU.NUCL., abducens nucleus; INF., inferior vestibular nucleus; LAT., lateral vestibular nucleus (of Deiters); Medial, medial vestibular nucleus; Super., superior vestibular nucleus; MLF, medial longitudinal fasciculus. Oculomotor subgroups: IO, inferior oblique muscle; IR, inferior rectus muscle; MR, medial rectus muscle; SR, superior rectus muscle; Troc. Nuc., trochlear nucleus.

glossopharyngeal nerve (IX) and to the dorsal motor nucleus and nucleus ambiguus of the vagus (X) in initiating vomiting. Other connections presumably also influence the motor cells of the ventral horn of the spinal cord which may become associated with posture during vomiting. Since this is a well-coordinated reflex, it is not to be doubted but that the vestibular cerebellar connections also play a role.

E. Clinical correlates.

1. Nystagmus is a term used for certain types of conjugate movements of the eyes such that the eyes may have a slow movement in one direction and

a fast movement in the opposite direction, when the body is rotated in an acceleratory manner. This is a response which may be induced in any normal person. The eye movements result from unequal stimulation of the vestibular cristae in the semicircular canals of the two sides which are in the same plane of rotation. This is due to the fact that acceleratory rotation induces a movement in the labyrinth which is not paralleled by the movement of the contained endolymph. Thus, during rotation, the fluid tends to move away from the receptor of one side (negative effect) and toward the equivalent receptor on the other side (positive effect). This imbalance of stimuli sets up reflex responses which provoke the alternating movements of the eyes. The quick-moving component of the alternate to-and-fro movements is toward the side of maximal (positive) stimulation.

a. Since nystagmus may normally be induced in a healthy person with intact receptors by rotatory or caloric stimuli, it holds that failure to induce these movements or an exaggeration of the normal response would be indicative of a pathologic state of the vestibular system. Further, the presence of nystagmoid movements without the use of appropriate stimuli, suggesting an inherent imbalance of stimuli at the receptors, would also imply disease.

b. Cerebellar nystagmus. This is probably not a true nystagmus, but an ataxia of the extraocular muscles. However, the close proximity of the vestibular nuclei may cause involvement of both components of the CNS in disease. Further, disease of the flocculonodular lobe of the cerebellum, with its intimate association with the vestibular nuclei, may provide for what could be a true cerebellar nystagmus. If the eye movements do not show well-defined slow and quick components and there is associated cerebellar disease, one may consider that the abnormal eye movements may simply be another form of cerebellar ataxia.

c. Peripheral nystagmus (disease at the level of the receptor) is of the horizontal-rotatory type with a quick component to the nonaffected side. There is vertigo, past-pointing, a tendency to fall and autonomic symptoms. It is transitory, implying that the vestibular nuclei can accommodate for the altered distribution of impulses.

d. Central nystagmus differs from the peripheral disease in that vertigo is almost absent and the other symptoms do not subside. It is usually related to disseminated sclerosis.

e. Optokinetic nystagmus can occur in any plane and is related to visual stimuli such as occur when watching a long line of poles pass by one after the other from the window of a fast-moving vehicle. An ocular nystagmus may also be present in persons with defective vision. This usually develops shortly after birth and is pendular in nature. This form probably represents a reflex attempt to increase the amount of information impinging on the retina.

f. Vertigo is a false sense of rotation of self or surrounding objects which may be induced by vestibular disease and is often associated with autonomic overactivity to produce nausea, vomiting, tachycardia and diarrhea.

167

g. Meniere's disease is associated with nausea, vertigo, vomiting, tinnitus and progressive deafness and is frequently associated with increased pressure of the endolymph in the membranous labyrinth.

h. Sea sickness is a transient disorder related to violent stimulation of the vestibular receptors which produce all the symptoms of vertigo.

Chapter 16

THE CEREBELLAR SYSTEM

The cerebellum is a structure which is intimately associated with the function of the motor system. Without the cerebellum, motor function decomposes into an uncoordinated state in which there is an inadequate control of muscle action such that the smooth performance of any motor response becomes jerky and uncertain. The gross appearance is of a tremor during movement (intention tremor), frequently termed ataxia.

Cerebellar function is based primarily on the acquisition of information from the body (spinocerebellar tracts) as to the position of the body parts,

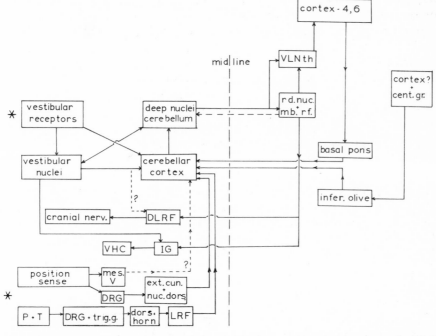

Fig. 111. A schematic illustration of the nuclear interconnections concerned with the cerebellar system. cent. gr., central grey of the mesencephalon; ext. cun., external cuneate nucleus; DLRF, dorsolateral reticular formation; dors. horn, dorsal horn of spinal cord and descending trigeminal nucleus; DRG, dorsal root ganglia; IG, intermediate grey of spinal cord; inf. olive, inferior olivary nucleus; LRF, ventrolateral reticular formation; mb. rf., midbrain reticular formation; mes. V, mesencephalic tract and nucleus of the trigeminal nerve; nuc. dors., nucleus dorsalis (of Clarke); P + T, pain and temperature receptors; rd. nuc., red nucleus; trig. g., ganglion of the trigeminal nerve; VHC, ventral horn motor neurons; VLNth, ventrolateral nucleus of the thalamus.

169

or information from the muscles of the face as to their relative position or degree of tension (via the mesencephalic tract and nucleus of the trigeminal nerve and as yet ill-defined central pathways), and on two levels of input from higher centers. There is first an input arising from the cerebral cortex which is relayed by the basal pontine nuclei to the contralateral cerebellar cortex. This path appears to relate to an intended motor act originating in the cortex and pertains to the nonstereotyped kind of motor action requiring fine movements of the extremities. The second input from higher centers originates in the central grey (mesencephalic) and other subcortical higher centers which are not too well-defined. It passes through the central tegmental fasciculus, and is relayed by the inferior olive to the contralateral cerebellar cortex. It is believed by some authors that influences arising in the basal ganglia are relayed to the cerebellum following a synapse in the central grey and that these pertain to cerebellar regulation of the more automatic sequences of motor function, such as arm swinging in quadrapedal progression. Thus, the spinal cord and trigeminal inputs provide information pertaining to position sense (unconscious proprioception), while the pontine and olivary relayed inputs from higher levels relate to intended motor functions. Based on these inputs the cerebellum is in a position to influence the intended motor function back via its relay through the red nucleus (and reticular formation) to the ventral anterior and ventrolateral nuclei of the thalamus, which in turn projects to the motor and premotor cortex. There are also direct cerebellar thalamic projections. The sequence of these connections is illustrated in Fig. 111. It should be noted that the influence of the cerebellar cortex on the proper synergic control of motor response is relayed from the cortex by the deep cerebellar nuclei (dentate, emboliform, globose and fastigial), and that the entering afferents from the spinal cord and pontine nuclei provide for collaterals which also terminate in these deep nuclei. It is suggested by experiments wherein the cerebellar cortex is removed, and from the results of neurosurgical removal of the cerebellar cortex in patients, that the resultant impairment of function is less if these deep nuclei are spared. This suggests that at least some part of the cerebellar regulatory function may be subserved by these deep nuclei.

A. Some idea of the major anatomical components of the cerebellum may be inferred from Fig. 112. Note that the cerebellum consists of a midline vermis which is coextensive with the laterally directed hemispheres, and that the hemisphere may be divided into a small anterior lobe rostral to the primary fissure and a large posterior lobe. There is further a phylogenetically old flocculonodular lobe which has close connections with the vestibular system.

B. The distribution of afferent inputs to the various regions of the cerebellum is illustrated in Fig. 113, which also provides some idea as to the topographic localization of the body parts within the cerebellum. Note that axial parts of

170

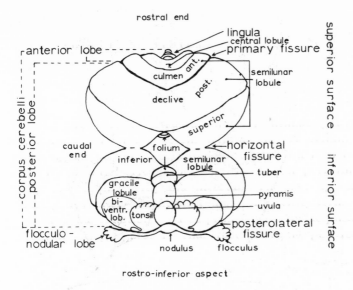

Fig. 112. A diagrammatic illustration of the anatomical components of the cerebellum.

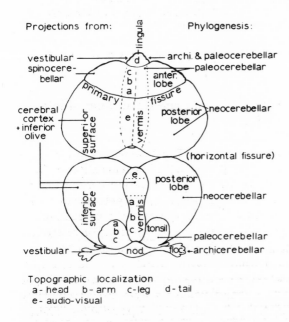

Fig. 113. A diagrammatic illustration of the components of the cerebellum in relation to phylogenetic age and sources of inputs.

171

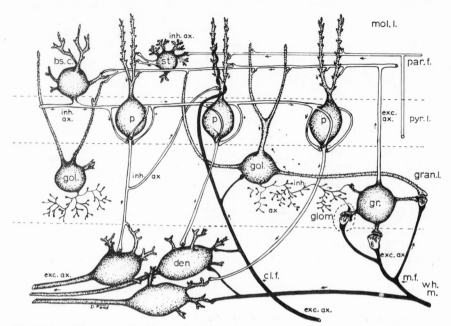

Fig. 114. A diagrammatic illustration (based on Eccles *et al.*, 1967) of the cellular components and connections within the cerebellar cortex. bs. c., basket cell; cl. f., climbing fiber; den, cells of the dentate nucleus; exc. ax., excitatory axon; glom., glomerulus; gol., Golgi cell; gr., granule cell; gran. l., granule cell layer; inh. ax., inhibitory axon; m. f., mossy fiber; mol. l., molecular layer; p, Purkinje cell; par. f., parallel fibers; pyr. l., Purkinje cell layer; st, stellate cell; wh. m., white matter.

the body are represented medially and that the appendicular parts are represented laterally.

C. The major cell types, the distribution of inputs and the manner of inter-action between cells is illustrated by Fig. 114.

D. Clinical correlations. Interference in cerebellar function as a result of vascular disease, tumor, multiple sclerosis, postsynaptic degeneration of the cerebellum, damage to the basal pontine nuclei or the efferent cerebellar tracts is characterized by the presence of tremor during the performance of a motor act. The tremor is ipsilateral to the lesion if it is in the cerebellar hemisphere, restricted to the trunk if the lesion is in the vermis, or restricted to an extremity if the lesion is sufficiently far lateral in the hemisphere.

1. Patients demonstrate a tremor (ataxia) in attempting to place the finger on the tip of the nose, which is not worsened when the eyes are closed. They have difficulty in running one heel down the shin of the opposite leg. There is difficulty in performing rapidly opposing movements (dysdiadochokinesia) and tonus of muscles may be reduced.

Chapter 17

DESCENDING SUPRASPINAL SYSTEMS

In this discussion the author has elected to continue the precedent established by Brodal (*Neurological Anatomy*) and to avoid referring to the motor
system as consisting of pyramidal and extrapyramidal systems. While there
are indeed motor systems descending from the cerebral cortex and from
various subcortical levels which effect motor responses, there are, in addition,
fibers running in the same pathway which terminate on cells of the nucleus
cuneatus and nucleus gracilis, in the sensory nuclei of the trigeminal nerve,
and on cells of the dorsal horn. There are, in addition, efferent impulses
relayed to the retina and inner ear receptors. All of these are believed to
influence the function of the sensory receptor elements and it is difficult to
fit these fiber projections directly into a motor system, even though their
fibers run with the motor pathways, and which, by influencing afferent systems,
may ultimately alter the motor system output.

A. Classically, neuroanatomists and neurologists have described a pyramidal
system and an extrapyramidal system. This dicotomy was based on early
observations by neurologists that lesions effecting the fibers that run through
the pyramids at the base of the medulla produce one class of symptoms as
compared with other motor disorders wherein the lesions are unrelated to the
fibers passing through the pyramids. If lesions of the fibers related to the
pyramids produce pyramidal tract disease of the motor system, those lesions
not in this fiber tract system which influence motor function should logically
produce an "extra" pyramidal disease. Included in this category were symptoms associated with lesions of the basal ganglia, substantia nigra and subthalamic nucleus. Presumably these structures would have to have a major
downstream projection to the spinal cord if they were to provide for a parallel
extrapyramidal motor system. Unfortunately, however, these subcortical
nuclei have very little in the way of a distal cord or lower brain stem projection.
The major efferent projection from the basal ganglia is from the medial
division of the globus pallidus which sends fibers to the ventral anterior and
ventrolateral nuclei of the thalamus, to the hypothalamus, the subthalamic
nucleus, the substantia nigra, the red nucleus, the reticular formation and the
inferior olive. While the rubro-olivoreticulospinal projection may provide for a
descending complex of fibers parallel to the pyramidal system to influence
the motor cell elements, the major projection from the pallidum is to the
thalamus which relays the influence of the striatum to the motor and premotor cortex in conjunction with its relay of the cerebellar influence. It thus

173

seems unlikely that the nuclei of the basal ganglia constitute a major locus of extrapyramidal influence on motor function. Rather, they seem to be part of a general motor system and to act in consort with the cerebellum to modulate the activity of the motor cortex. If one were therefore to describe what the components are of an extrapyramidal system, that is a system which influences motor responses and which parallels the pyramidal system, one would have to consider the following pathways, including their cells of origin.

1. Vestibulospinal tracts (medial and lateral).

2. Tectospinal tract, from the superior colliculus.

3. Interstitiospinal tract, arising from the interstitial nucleus of Cajal in the mesencephalon.

4. Fibers from the nuclei of the raphe to the spinal cord.

5. Reticulospinal tracts.

B. The so-called pyramidal system has been observed to arise from cells in area 4 of the motor cortex, area 6 of the premotor cortex, areas 3, 1 and 2 of the primary sensory cortex and from areas 40 and 43, as well as from the supplementary motor area on the medial surface of the hemisphere (above the gyrus cinguli extending forward from the leg region of primary motor cortex). By the time it enters the pyramids at the base of the medulla, it contains only about 1000 000 fibers, many having left the tract system to terminate on neurons of the cranial nerve motor neurons (corticobulbar fibers). This component may reasonably be called the direct corticospinal-cortico-bulbar pathway. Other axons arising from the cortex only attain the level of the basal ganglia. A parallel fiber pathway system arising from the same cortical areas as the direct pathway and which also passes through the internal capsule may be termed the indirect corticospinal pathway. This consists of a corticorubro- and a corticoreticulospinal projection system which also influences the activity of motor cells in the ventral horn of the spinal cord.

1. In the distribution of fibers of this system, it has been observed that those fibers destined to innervate motor neurons associated with the extremities all cross through the pyramidal decussation to supply the contra-lateral side. Those destined for axial musculature in general supply the neurons of both sides. This also applies in general to the nuclei of the motor type cranial nerves, with the following exceptions. Those neurons which will innervate the lower two-thirds of the face (VII) are innervated only by the

174

contralateral cortex. The same has also been said to apply to the neurons of the hypoglossal and accessory nuclei on the basis of clinical observations, but this is open to discussion.

2. The fibers leave the cerebral cortex and pass through the posterior limb of the internal capsule without a sharply defined topographic localization. They then pass through the medial two-thirds of the pes pedunculi with the fibers for the face being most medial. These are followed in turn by fibers for arm and trunk, with the fibers destined to innervate the leg being most lateral. These fibers then break up into a number of fascicles in the pons and then recoalesce in the pyramids. At the medullar-spinal cord junction about 85% of the fibers decussate to enter the lateral funiculus of the spinal cord. The remaining 15% descend ipsilaterally, mostly in the ventral funiculus. This latter group rarely descends below the thoracic cord and many of its fibers will cross through the anterior white commissure of the cord before terminating. Most of these will terminate on intercalated (internuncial) cells which then relay the signals to the motor neurons. Some of the uncrossed fibers pass in the lateral corticospinal tract and terminate on internuncials innervating motor neurons ipsilaterally. During its course through the mesencephalon, pons and medulla, numerous fibers leave the tract to innervate cranial nerve motor neurons. It seems unlikely that this innervation is mediated by an internuncial neuron, but is direct, as are probably most of the terminals for innervation of the hand. This pathway is what may be referred to as the direct corticospinal-corticobulbar pathway. Fibers within the indirect corticospinal tract system lose their association with the direct corticospinal system at the level of the midbrain where they terminate on cells of the red nucleus or reticular formation. This system remains anatomically disassociated from the direct system until reaching the level of the spinal cord. From this level caudally, the corticorubrospinal system mingles with the lateral corticospinal tract and many of the reticulospinal tract fibers are just adjacent.

3. Some corticofugal fibers do not enter into the primary motor pathway, but pass in close relationship to it to terminate on cells of the pons for relay to the contralateral cerebellar cortex. These corticopontine fibers arise from the frontal, temporal, parietal and occipital cortex, pass through the internal capsule and are either medial or lateral to the motor pathway in the midbrain.

4. The neomotor direct pathways, including the corticopontine relay to the cerebellum, and a relay involving the striatum, are illustrated schematically in Fig. 115.

5. The classical nuclear groups of what has been called the extrapyramidal system are those cells of the basal ganglia, substantia nigra and subthalamic nucleus. However, as previously indicated, the anatomical connections of these neurons suggest that their role is primarily in influencing the activity of

175

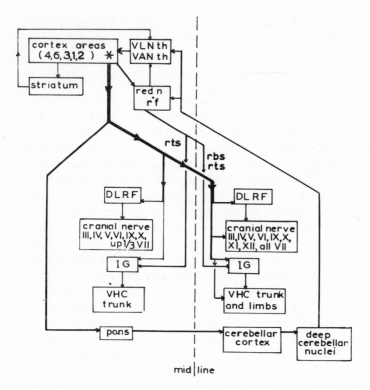

MOTOR PATHWAYS
CORTICOSPINAL   CORTICOBULBAR

Fig. 115. A schematic diagram illustrating the components of the direct and indirect corticospinal systems, including those connections made with the cerebellum and through the striatum which may influence the function of the motor system. DLRF, dorsolateral reticular formation; IG, intermediate grey (locus for internuncial cells); rbs, rubrospinal tract; rf, reticular formation; red n, red nucleus; rts, reticulospinal tract; VANth, ventral anterior nucleus of thalamus; VHC, ventral horn motor neuron; VLNth, ventrolateral nucleus of thalamus. The direct motor pathway commences at the motor cortex and is relayed to the motor cells of the spinal cord and motor cranial nerve nuclei through cells of the dorsolateral reticular formation or intermediate grey. The indirect motor pathway reaches the level of the spinal cord via a relay in the red nucleus or reticular formation. Observe that the crossed cortical projection (large heavy line) has direct connections on cranial nerve and spinal cord motor neurons, as well as indirect connections. These probably arise mainly from the giant pyramidal cells (Betz cells) of layer 5 of the motor cortex (area 4). Most of the terminals of this sort would appear to be in relation to facial innervation and to a lesser extent the hand.

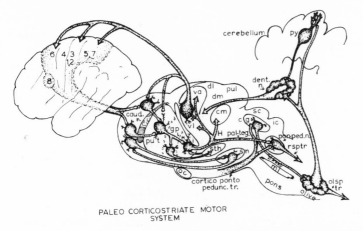

PALEO CORTICOSTRIATE MOTOR
SYSTEM

Fig. 116. A schematic illustration of the components making up the paleocorticostriate part of the motor system. caud. n., caudate nucleus; cg, central grey of mesencephalon; cm, centrum medianum of thalamus; dent. n., dentate nucleus of cerebellum; dm, dorsomedial nucleus of thalamus; gp (1 + m), medial and lateral divisions of the globus pallidus; H, tegmental field of Forel; ic, internal capsule; ml, medial lemniscus; oc, optic chiasm; olsptr, olivospinal tract; pal-teg., pallidotegmental tract; pon-ped. n., pontopeduncular nucleus; put, putamen; pul, pulvinar; py, Purkinje cell of cerebellar cortex; rsptr, reticulospinal tract; sc, superior colliculus; ic, inferior colliculus; sn, substantia nigra; sth, subthalamic nucleus; va, ventral anterior nucleus of thalamus; vl, ventrolateral nucleus of thalamus; zi, zona incerta.

cortical neurons. In the case of the substantia nigra, its primary role appears to be at the level of the caudate nucleus (Fig. 116). These nuclear groups do, however, have terminations on the mesencephalic central grey, the reticular formation and the pontopeduncular nuclei which may give rise to a small group of descending fibers which influence the function of the lower motor neuron. It should be noted that the cortical areas which project to the cortico-spinal and corticobulbar systems are essentially the same as those giving rise to fibers innervating the basal ganglia and indirect corticospinal systems. Indeed, these projections may come from an even greater cortical area.

C. Motor neurons.

1. The upper motor neuron. This cell is generally considered to be in layer 5 of the cortex which gives rise to the corticofugal fiber system which projects the motor signal to effector neurons which innervate muscles, etc. However, other subcortical neurons whose axons project to motor nuclei may also be considered "upper" in relation to the final neurons of the circuit.

2. Lower motor neurons. These are the final common pathway cells described by Sherrington, and are the cells which directly innervate the musculature.

3. Internuncial neurons. The influence of the upper motor neuron on the lower motor neuron is generally considered to be mediated via an internuncial neuron, though there are instances wherein the relationship between the two levels of motor neuron is direct. These direct connections are probably all mediated via the giant pyramidal (Betz) neurons.

D. Clinical correlations.

1. Diseases of the upper motor neurons. These are caused by any process which interrupts the corticofugal fiber system on its way to the internuncial neurons and the lower motor neurons. The resultant symptoms are typical and related apparently to the fact that the lower motor neurons are still functional and influenced by other lower subcortical motor components. The symptoms associated with disease of the upper motor neurons represent a composite effect of an injury effecting neurons of cortical origin and those of subcortical origin wherein the lower motor neurons no longer receive innervation from that part of the system which elicits voluntary motor response but are still subject to influences derived from a spinal or brain stem level. These are:

a. Increase in tonus of the muscles. This is believed to be due to an influence on the functional state of the efferent system by various brain stem systems. Deep tendon reflexes are accordingly increased.

b. There is a development of spasticity after an initial period of flaccidity shortly after the lesion occurs. This is manifested by an over-contraction of the antigravity muscles (paralysis in extension in the legs and paralysis in flexion of the arms: clasp-knife reflex).

c. Electrical activity of muscles is maintained.

d. Superficial reflexes such as the abdominal and cremasteric are lost.

e. The plantar reflex (plantar flexion of the big toe when the sole of the foot is stroked from the heel toward the toe) is lost and replaced by dorsi-flexion of the big toe and fanning of the other toes (Babinski toe sign).

f. Ankle clonus.

2. Diseases of the lower motor neurons involve destruction of the nerve cells or their fibers which directly innervate the muscles. Thus, no neural influence can reach the muscles. Symptoms are characterized by:

a. Loss of all electrical activity in muscles.

b. Loss of all reflex activity.

c. Flaccidity of the muscles at first which is eventually replaced by contractures.

d. Atrophy of the muscles with fasciculations during the period of developing atrophy.

e. Such processes may result from poliomyelitis, vascular accident to the spinal cord, traumatic injury to the cord, compression of the ventral roots or a chronic degenerative disease such as amyotrophic lateral sclerosis, which involves both the corticospinal system and the motor neurons.

3. Alternating hemiplegias. These occur at sites where the descending corticospinal system passes in close proximity to an exiting motor nerve.

a. Upper alternating hemiplegia occurs with lesions involving the basis pedunculi and the exiting fibers of the oculomotor nerve. There is a contralateral spastic paralysis of the extremities and a flaccid lower motor neuron paralysis of the muscles innervated by the IIIrd cranial nerve.

b. Middle alternating hemiplegia occurs at the level of the exiting fibers of the abducens nerve and again causes contralateral spastic paralysis of extremities with an associated ipsilateral lower motor neuron paralysis involving the abducens nerve distribution to the lateral rectus muscle of the eye.

c. Lower alternating hemiplegia occurs at the level of the exiting hypoglossal nerve fibers. Again there is a crossed spastic paralysis of extremities and ipsilateral flaccid paralysis of the tongue muscle.

4. There is another category of diseases, usually classified as being extrapyramidal, but which in reality are due to diseases of subcortical nuclear regions whose major neural impact is on the cerebral cortex. In some of these diseases the cortex is also involved.

a. Parkinsonism primarily involves disease of the substantia nigra, though there are also said to be changes in the globus pallidus (this may be indirect and due to overactivity). Symptoms consist of:

(i) Rigidity of the musculature.

(ii) Paucity of facial expression.

(iii) Tremor at rest with a frequency of 6 to 10 per second.

(iv) A pill-rolling movement of the fingers and gaping movements of the mouth.

(v) Excessive sweating and secretion of sebum.

(vi) Deep tendon reflexes are depressed, and there is cog-wheeling and resistance to movement.

(vii) The disease has been associated with encephalitis, arteriosclerosis, nigrostriatal degeneration, drugs such as reserpine, infectious diseases, manganese, carbon monoxide and carbon disulfide poisoning.

(viii) It has been treated surgically by thalamotomy of the ventrolateral nucleus and by treatment with L-DOPA. The latter drug becomes converted to dopamine within the caudate nucleus and is believed to be effective because it serves as a therapy for replacement of the dopamine lost from the caudate following lesions of the substantia nigra.

b. Dystonia musculorum deformans (torsion dystonia) is a disease in which there are dystonic movements producing abnormal postures. The disease may be inherited as an autosomal dominant.

(i)   Neuronal losses have been observed in the putamen, caudate nucleus, dentate nucleus, substantia nigra and thalamus.

(ii) Some relief of symptoms has been achieved with Valium and antihistamines. Thalamotomy of the ventrolateral nucleus of the thalamus has been said to produce favorable results in some cases.

(iii) Spasmodic torticollis. This is a limited form of dystonia confined to the neck musculature.

c. Chorea. This is a disease characterized by brief, purposeless involuntary movements, primarily of the face and extremities. Facial grimacing is common. There is decreased tone and generalized weakness.

(i) In Sydenham's chorea there is often an associated history of rheumatic fever. Lesions appear to be related to areas of arteritis producing neuronal losses in the cortex, basal ganglia, brain stem and cerebellum.

(ii) Chlorpromazine has been used with some success for treatment and can be withdrawn if side effects characteristic of other extrapyramidal diseases develop.

d. Athetosis. This is a disease process wherein there are writhing movements of the extremities.

(i) It appears related to striatopallidal damage secondary to anoxic encephalopathy at or shortly after birth.

e. Huntington's chorea is an inherited form of choreo-athetosis of unknown etiology. It is carried as an autosomal dominant and is marked by a complete loss of the small neurons of the caudate nucleus and putamen with accompanying reactive gliosis. Neuronal loss also occurs to a greater or lesser degree in the cortex, subthalamic nucleus, dentate nucleus and cerebellar cortex.

(i) Antidepressant drugs or psychic energizers such as the monoamine oxidase inhibitors have had some success in treatment. Reserpine suppresses many of the abnormal movements. Other patients have responded to drugs of the phenathiazine group or to Valium.

f. Hemiballismus. This is a term used to describe the violent flinging movements of the extremities which occur subsequent to damage of the contralateral subthalamic nucleus or to its connection with the globus pallidus.

(i) It may result from arteriosclerosis, meningovascular syphilis or be the consequence of viral encephalitis or granulomatous inflammation.

(ii) It has been treated with some success with Valium.

5. The diseases of the subcortical nuclear groups which lead to abnormal movements may be loosely grouped into two classes. There is a hypokinetic type of patient who is characterized by the Parkinsonian patient where there is a paucity of movement. Then there are the hyperkinesias where there is excessive, uncontrolled movement. These may be schematized in the manner illustrated in Fig. 117. In athetosis there is a continuity of movement, but

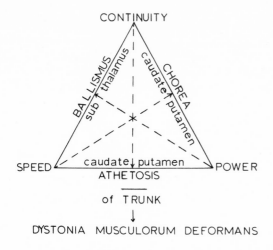

CONTINUITY

BALLISMUS
sub thalamus

CHOREA
caudate putamen

SPEED   caudate putamen   POWER
ATHETOSIS

of TRUNK

DYSTONIA MUSCULORUM DEFORMANS

Fig. 117. A schematic illustration of certain disorders of the corticostriate component of the motor system. The names of the disorders are given along the sides of the triangle and a word which characterizes the nature of the movement is indicated at the opposite angle of the triangle. The major site of pathologic disorder for each of these motor disorders is given on the inside of the triangle. The particular disorders related to the triangle are disorders of the extremities in which there is excessive movement (hyperkinesia). A related problem, but restricted to the trunk, is dystonia.

without speed or power. In chorea there is speed without continuity or power, while in ballismus there is power without continuity or speed. All of these movements refer to the appendages. Comparable hyperkinetic movements occur in the trunk as dystonia deformans or as spasmodic torticollis.

Chapter 18

INTER-RELATIONSHIP BETWEEN SENSORY AND MOTOR SYSTEMS

It becomes apparent as one studies the nervous system that there is a considerable degree of interaction between the various areas of the brain. The sort of projections of information which eventually involve large parts of the CNS may be illustrated by the various types of inter-regional interaction which occur following activation of receptors in either the retina or the cochlea (Fig. 118). In this instance both are provided with connections to various reflex levels of the brain stem, to areas of associational cortex and by pathways which connect eventually with the motor system to induce coordinative movements of the body. While it is not yet clear that all these components may respond from each stimulus input, it is clear from anatomical and physiological studies that the substrata for such interaction is available to mammalian forms.

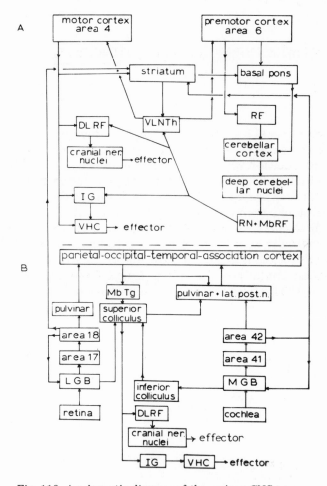

Fig. 118. A schematic diagram of the various CNS components which may become involved in the response to a visual or auditory signal arising from the primary receptor organ. DLRF, dorsolateral reticular formation; IG, intermediate grey matter of spinal cord; lat. post. n., posterolateral nucleus of thalamus; LGB, lateral geniculate body; MbTg, midbrain tegmentum; MGB, medial geniculate body; RF, reticular formation; RN + MbRF, red nucleus + midbrain reticular formation; VHC, ventral horn motor neuron.

Chapter 19

THE OLFACTORY AND LIMBIC SYSTEMS

An extremely important component of the CNS is the limbic system with its associated olfactory input, which is indirect. A wide variety of ablation and stimulation studies on numerous species have led us to understand that this phylogenetically old portion of the CNS is related to responses dealing with sexual, feeding and stress behavior. In affecting these behavioral responses, it is intimately associated with the hypothalamus and the endocrine system. An analysis of the various experimental findings may lead to some frustration because of the numerous contradictions in results between different species or experimental procedures. However, one may summarize these findings as dealing with two major types of behavior. First, there are those responses which deal with the maintenance of the species. These of course deal with all

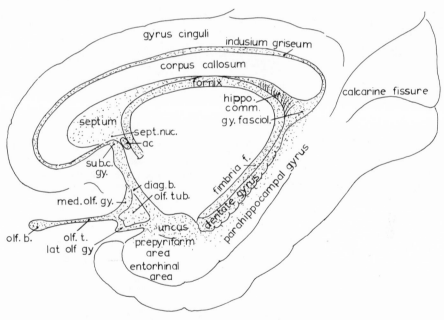

Fig. 119. A diagrammatic illustration of the telencephalic components of the limbic system. ac, anterior commissure; diag. b., diagonal band of Broca; fimbria f., fimbria of fornix; gy. fasciol., gyrus fasciolaris; hippo. comm., hippocampal commissure; lat olf gy, lateral olfactory gyrus; med. olf. gy., medial olfactory gyrus; olf. b., olfactory bulb; olf. t., olfactory tract; olf. tub., olfactory tubercle; sept. nuc., septal nucleus; sub. c. gy., subcallosal gyrus. Stippled areas indicate the macroscopic components of the rhinencephalon.

the various types of reproductive behavior (mate searching, courtship, copulatory responses, nesting, etc.). Second, there are those responses which deal with the preservation of the individual. These would include the various types of behavior involved with the search for food and defense against various enemy species or predators.

A. The anatomical components of the limbic and olfactory systems occupied a large part of the CNS of primitive species. In man, however, this part of the CNS has been overshadowed by more recent phylogenetic elements. The major telencephalic components of the limbic and olfactory systems are illustrated in Fig. 119. Not shown are the primary olfactory neurons which project from the olfactory epithelium to the mitral cells of the olfactory bulb and the diencephalic components. The hippocampus, a major cortical region of the limbic system, is also not shown as it is situated lateral to the dentate gyrus.

B. Afferent olfactory projections as indicated by Allison. The major nuclear terminations of the mitral cells in the olfactory bulb are indicated in Fig. 120.

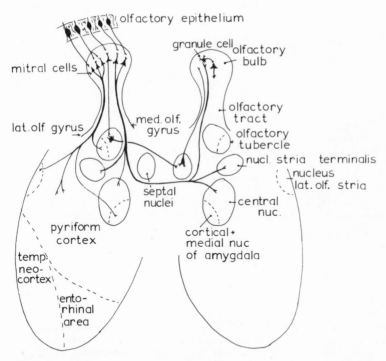

Fig. 120. A diagrammatic illustration (after Allison) of the afferent olfactory projections. med. olf. gyrus, medial olfactory gyrus; lat. olf gyrus, lateral olfactory gyrus; lat. olf. stria, lateral olfactory stria.

186

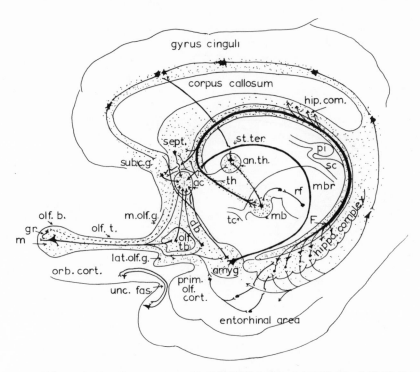

Fig. 121. A diagrammatic representation of the afferent and associative connections of the limbic system. ac, anterior commissure; amyg, amygdala; an. th., anterior nucleus of thalamus; db, diagonal band of Broca; F, fornix; gr, granule cell; hip. com., hippocampal commissure; lat. olf. g., lateral olfactory gyrus; m, mitral cell; mb, mammillary body; mbr, midbrain reticular formation; m. olf. g., medial olfactory gyrus; olf. b., olfactory bulb; olf. t., olfactory tract; olf. tb., olfactory tubercle; orb. cort., orbital cortex; pi, pineal gland; prim. olf. cort., primary olfactory cortex; rf, reticular formation; sc, superior colliculus; sept., septal nuclei; st. ter, stria terminalis; sub. c. g., subcallosal gyrus; tc, tuber cinereum; th, thalamus; unc. fas., uncinate fasciculus.

Note that there are no connections which are made directly to the hippocampus. Any olfactory input to this extremely important structure of the limbic system must be accomplished indirectly. The precise nature of such a pathway is still uncertain.

C. The limbic system contains within its multiplicity of cortical and nuclear structures a wide variety of interconnections which in some way subserve the various functions of the system. The various afferent and associative connections are illustrated in Fig. 121, while the major efferent components are illustrated in Fig. 122. Some degree of overlap may be noted. However, it is the connections shown in the latter figure which provide for the limbic projection to lower brain stem regions and presumably may be involved in some of the behavioral responses of the organism.

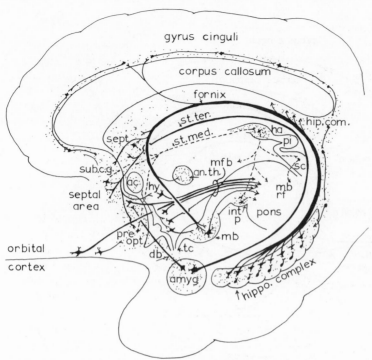

Fig. 122. A diagrammatic illustration of the efferent connections of the rhinencephalon. ac, anterior commissure; an. th., anterior thalamic nucleus; db, diagonal band of Broca; ha, habenular nucleus; hip. com., hippocampal commissure; hippo. complex, hippocampal complex; hy, hypothalamus; int p, interpeduncular nucleus; mb, mammillary body; mbrf, midbrain reticular formation; mfb, medial forebrain bundle; pi, pineal gland; pre opt, preoptic area; sept, septum pellucidum; st. med., stria medullaris; st. ter., stria terminalis; sub. c. g., subcallosal gyrus; tc, tuber cinereum.

1. One type of connection not illustrated relates to the impact of the preoptic and septal areas of the hypothalamus. These would appear to be in a position to influence the releasing factors of the hypothalamus which then in turn regulate the adenohypophysis. Such connections presumably may account for the effect of fear in suppressing menstrual cycles in humans or the spontaneous abortions which occur among pregnant rats in the presence of foreign males or the urine of such males. By other pathways a sensory input derived from changes in the external environment (i.e. seasons) may impinge on these same hypothalamic areas to induce migratory and seasonal reproductive behavior. Similarly, the tactile stimuli arising from the vagina in reflex-ovulating animals influence the hypothalamus via spinal afferents to regulate adenohypophyseal gonadotropic hormones. Another influence which appears dependent on the septal-preoptic area, hypothalamus interconnections, relates to the effects of such stresses as anxiety or tension on the functions of the vagus nerve.

D. Clinical considerations.

1. Damage to the olfactory bulb or tract leads to anosmias. These may result from fractures in the region of the cribriform plate, and meningiomas of the olfactory groove or suprasellar region and may give rise to unilateral or bilateral olfactory loss, depending on location. Diseases of the frontal lobe (gliomas or abscesses) may sooner or later influence the olfactory bulb or tract due to pressure.

2. Lesions of the temporal lobe.
   a. Homonymous quadrantic hemianopsias frequently result due to damage to the lower fibers of the optic radiations.
   b. Bilateral temporal lobe lesions involving the hippocampus lead to losses of recent memory and progressive dementia. Old memory usually remains intact and there seems to be little loss of personality or general intelligence. The degree of memory loss seems to vary with the extent of hippocampal damage. Unilateral damage to the hippocampus, uncus and amygdaloid nucleus has not been reported to cause any severe psychological impairment. It is, however, difficult to relate the hippocampus specifically to memory in man since in no reported case has the damage been restricted to the hippocampus. Experiments with animals in which the hippocampus and amygdala have been bilaterally destroyed have lead to a description of the losses of function by Klüver and Bucy which has come to be called the Klüver-Bucy syndrome. There is:
      (i)   Visual agnosia.
      (ii) Orality — virtually every object seen is placed in the mouth.
      (iii) Hypermetamorphosis — a tendency to pay attention to every visual stimulus.
      (iv) A depression of emotional response or taming.
      (v)   An increase in sexual activity.
      (vi) A change in dietary habits (in monkeys).
To what extent these phenomena occur in man is challenged by some neurologists who claim that this syndrome complex is rarely encountered in its totality in patients. What has been apparent is a memory deficit and some increase in sexual activity in males, which is hormone dependent.
   c. Temporal lobe epilepsy originating from disease processes of the temporal lobe is often associated with special kinds of consciousness. Thus, among the initial symptoms there may be an acoustic aura or an olfactory sensation (uncinate fits). Other cases describe complex psychic experiences as an aura. It is common during the attack that the patient is unresponsive and there may be some loss of understanding even if motor and sensory functions remain intact. This type of epilepsy is often termed psychomotor.

Chapter 20

THE AUTONOMIC NERVOUS SYSTEM

The highest level of the autonomic system (Fig. 123) within the CNS is the hypothalamus. It is influenced by hormonal, environmental and psychic factors which impinge on it either directly or which are mediated through connections with the limbic cortex, preoptic area and amygdala. Lower autonomic centers in the midbrain, pontine and medullary reticular formation are then activated by a multisynaptic relay arising from within the hypothalamus. This multisynaptic relay continues into the spinal cord to terminate on preganglionic autonomic cells at that level as well.

A. Parasympathetic component (cholinergic fibers). This is the craniosacral division and consists of a series of preganglionic neurons associated with the 3rd, 7th, 9th and 10th cranial nerves. These neurons give off long preganglionic axons which terminate on postganglionic neurons in the walls of the organs innervated. The humoral product released is acetylcholine (cholinergic neurons). A similar situation exists in the sacral component where preganglionics with long nerve fibers arise from the 2nd, 3rd and 4th sacral nerves and pass via the nervi erigentes to synapse finally on postganglionic cells with short axons within the walls of the organ innervated.

B. The sympathetic division (adrenergic fibers peripherally). This system arises from the thoracolumbar level from spinal segments T_1 to L_2 or L_3. In distinction from the parasympathetic system, the preganglionic fibers are short relative to the postganglionic fibers. The preganglionic fibers pass for a short distance with the ventral root fibers and spinal nerves and then leave the spinal nerve to terminate in neurons in paravertebral ganglia. The fibers which leave the spinal nerves are heavily myelinated and hence are called the white rami. The fibers leaving the postganglionic neurons are very poorly myelinated and thus are termed grey rami. The transmitter substance released by the preganglionic sympathetic neurons is acetylcholine, while the postganglionic neurons release norepinephrine (adrenergic neurons). (Note that the sympathetic innervation of the adrenal medulla is by preganglionic fibers and there are no postganglionic units. The adrenergic transmitter component of a postganglionic nerve in this instance then is the hormone liberated by the adrenal medulla itself to induce a widespread blood-borne effect.)

1. Since there are no white rami arising from the spinal cord in cervical and lower lumbar and sacral levels, the postganglionic cells within the sympathetic

191

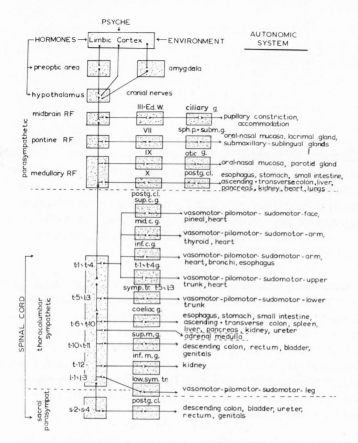

Fig. 123. A schematic outline of the units comprising the autonomic system. ciliary g., ciliary ganglion; coeliac g., coeliac ganglion; inf. c. g., inferior cervical ganglion; inf. m.g., inferior mesenteric ganglion; l, lumbar segment of cord; low. symp. tr., lower sympathetic trunk; mid. c.g., middle cervical ganglion; otic g., otic ganglion; postg. cl., postganglionic cells; RF, reticular formation; s, sacral level of the cord; sph. p + subm. g., sphenopalatine + submandibular ganglia; sup. c. g., superior cervical ganglion; sup. m. g., superior mesenteric ganglion; symp. tr., sympathetic trunk; t, thoracic segment of cord; III-Ed. W., Edinger and Westphal nucleus of the oculomotor nerve; VII, secretory nucleus of the facial nerve; IX, secretory nucleus of the glossopharyngeal nerve; X, dorsal motor nucleus of the vagus nerve.

ganglionic trunk at these levels are innervated by fibers which either descend or ascend to their levels via the sympathetic trunk. Thus, the cervical sympathetic postganglionic neurons are innervated by preganglionic neurons in the first four thoracic cord segments. These fibers then ascend through the sympathetic trunk to the appropriate levels. Sympathetic ganglia in the pelvic region are in turn supplied by preganglionics arising from the lowest thoracic segment and the upper lumbar segments.

192

2. Many of the so-called grey rami return immediately to the segmental spinal nerves at all levels and are distributed with them, supplying vasomotor, pilomotor and sudomotor fibers to the appropriate structures in the skin.

3. Preganglionics from the 5th thoracic segment to the 2nd or 3rd lumbar segment also provide for white rami which by-pass the ganglia of the sympathetic trunk to terminate on postganglionic cells in the coeliac, superior mesenteric and inferior mesenteric ganglia. Axons from cells in these ganglia are then distributed to the visceral organs via the splanchnic nerves.

C. Clinical considerations.

1. Lesions within the hypothalamus may produce:
   a. Diabetes insipidus.
   b. Disturbances in heat regulation.
   c. Vasomotor disturbances.
   d. Sleep disturbances (hypersomnia with posterior hypothalamic lesions).
   e. Dystrophia adiposogenitalis (with lesions in the tuberal nuclei and ventromedial nucleus).
   f. Hemorrhages and ulcerations of the alimentary canal.
   g. Horner's syndrome has been reported to occur with hypothalamic lesions.
   h. Hypothalamic lesions may also impinge on the optic chiasm or tracts to produce visual changes.

2. Lesions of the pons and medulla may interrupt the descending multi-synaptic autonomic path to preganglionic neurons of the lower brain stem and cord, abolishing autonomic reflexes below the level of the lesions. Thus, there may be anhidrosis, lack of pilomotor activity and vasodilation ipsilaterally. Horner's syndrome is usually apparent (constricted pupil with a dry flushed face on the side of the lesion). These all become less severe with time.

3. Lesions in the spinal cord, particularly from the 1st thoracic to the 2nd or 3rd lumbar level may be associated with segment to the 2nd or 3rd lumbar or sudomotor disturbances. Lesions in sacral level of the cord may lead to a paralyzed nonemptying bladder until distension is severe, when a little urine will be voided, but without emptying the bladder. There is also a loss of the ability to have an erection or ejaculation in the male. At the T_1-T_4 level there will also probably be Horner's syndrome.

4. Lesions of the peripheral ganglia may also occur with symptoms related to the ganglia involved.

5. Raynaud's disease. This is a disease more commonly found in women in which there are increases in vasomotor activity (constriction), particularly in the peripheral parts of the body. It is aided by sympathectomy.

6. Hirschsprung's disease (megacolon) appears to be due to congenital absence of, or inflammatory damage to, the myenteric plexus resulting in a tonus-depressing effect from the sympathetic supply from the coeliac ganglion to cause a localized enlargement of the bowel.

Chapter 21

CHANGES IN THE NERVOUS SYSTEM ASSOCIATED WITH MATURATION
AND AGING

The time of onset of age changes in the nervous system is difficult to relate
to a particular age. Furthermore, species differences have made it difficult to
utilize subprimate data in relation to man. At one time it was thought that
neurons were lost very rapidly (1000/hour), starting at birth. However, more
recent studies of Brody (1955) and Tomash (1971) have not verified this.
Brody's data indicate no real loss at least up until 21 years. There is, however,
a decrease in the cell population density as cell processes grow and push cells
further apart. On the other hand, the granular cells of layers II and IV of the
cerebral cortex do show a real decrease in number and are only rarely seen
between 70 and 95 years. Neuronal loss is most marked in the temporal lobe
and least in visual cortex. Thus, while cell loss is not as dramatic as previously
believed, some does occur and is most apparent in the very elderly. With aging,
there is also an increase in glial elements. What is also clear from numerous
studies of the brain in a wide variety of mammals is that there are maturational
changes which are prominent in the earlier phases which are probably of
greater significance than some of the changes related to true aging. While these
growth and maturational changes are determined primarily by the genetic
endowment of the individual, they are also influenced by hormonal, nutritional and environmental factors.

A. Maturational changes.

  1. Morphological.
     a. Studies with rats and other experimental animals have demonstrated
that there are marked increases in cell size with the development of longer and
more branched dendritic processes and axonal collaterals which occur postnatally. This serves to decrease nerve cell population density by pushing the
cells further apart. Similar observations have been made on man. These growth
and maturational changes have been shown by Eayrs to be extremely dependent on thyroid hormone and an adequate protein diet during the early developmental phase. Deficiency of either in experimental animals leads to
permanent retardation in the morphological development of the neurons.
Early postnatal nutritional deficiencies in rats have also been observed by
Balázs to produce a permanent deficit in cell number. Spinal cord and brain
stem neurons in rats appear more mature in relation to size and Nissl substance at an earlier date than cortical neurons.
     b. The proliferation of granule cells in the cerebellum, hippocampus and

olfactory cortex continues for some time after birth in all mammalian forms yet studied. This seems of particular importance in the cerebellum where the cells of the external granule cell layer not only continue to divide and eventually migrate into the inner granule cell layer, but give rise to the stellate and basket cells of the molecular layer of the cerebellar cortex.

c. Glial proliferation, particularly of oligodendroglial cells, occurs very markedly after birth, coinciding with the period of rapid myelinization. (Central myelin formation is dependent on the wrapping of oligodendroglial processes around axons.)

d. During this period of growth of cell processes and myelinization, there is a decrease in the size of the extracellular space as seen by electron microscopy. This is paralleled by an absolute decrease in water per unit volume and by a relative percent decrease in water per unit volume which is due as much to the increase in brain solids (protein, RNA and myelin) as to the decrease in extracellular space.

e. Synaptic structures become more numerous per unit area with the growth of the dendritic arborizations. The complexity of the synaptic substructure also increases during maturation.

f. Mitochondrial profiles have been observed to become more numerous during the period of rapid myelinization. Thus, it would seem that this increase may be associated with the marked increase in glial cells rather than with an increase in neuronal volume and size. Since thyroid-hormone responsive protein synthesis in neonates is dependent on mitochondria, these structures also appear significant in the period of rapid postnatal protein synthesis in neurons and in the total CNS. Finally, the association of both anaerobic and aerobic glycolytic enzyme systems with the mitochondria indicate further the importance of these organelles for the viability of neurons and glia.

g. Myelinization proceeds very rapidly just after birth. In man the most rapid period is during the first year to 18 months although myelinization may not be complete before 21 years of age. Phylogenetically older systems (reticulospinal, vestibulospinal tracts, central tegmental fasciculus, etc.) are more myelinated at birth than such newer systems as the cortical spinal system.

h. Ventricular dimensions increase during maturation as the size of the brain increases. However, while this overall increase in size is progressing, there is a counter effect due to the myelinization of the axons which are just subjacent to the ependyma in many areas of the ventricles which tends to reduce the overall size in proportion to the rest of the brain.

2. Influence of hormones. As previously indicated, thyroid hormone is essential during the early developmental stages of the brain. More recent studies suggest that thyroid hormone acts not only to stimulate growth and proliferation of neurons, but that it eventually also pushes neurons from the

proliferative to the differentiative stage. Thyroid hormone and estrogens have, on the other hand, been shown experimentally to stimulate myelinization. Conversely, thyroid deficiency leads to a 30% reduction in the dry weight of myelin in 43-day-old rats.

Corticosterone administration to experimental animals has been observed to delay the decrease in ventricular size associated with myelinization of the adjacent nerve fibers in mice, suggesting that the corticoid may inhibit myelin formation. The adrenal gland has also been linked to the synthesis of glycerol phosphate dehydrogenase in rats in that adrenalectomy depresses synthesis of the enzyme. Synthesis returns to normal when cortisol is provided to the animal. Corticosteroid (cortisol acetate) treatment in excess of normal to neonatal rats has further been shown to interfere with the normal postnatal brain mitotic activity leading to an overall decrease in cell numbers. Thus, while thyroid hormones appear to push neurons toward differentiation, cortisol depresses development of cells by inhibiting mitotic activity.

Testosterone and growth hormones have also been observed to have an anabolic effect in neural tissue. Testosterone has an additional effect in that it converts the hypothalamus into the noncyclic type during the early critical period just after birth in most mammals. Males lacking this hormonal influence would continue to possess hypothalamic structures which would permit the type of cyclic pituitary function which supports normal female ovarian and menstrual cycles. Newborn female rats treated with testosterone develop a male type of hypothalamus which fails to support cyclic pituitary function and leads to an anovulatory cycle. The presence or absence of testosterone in this early differentiative phase also influences subsequent sex behaviour in experimental animals (rats, hamsters, etc.).

3. Enzyme changes.

a. It has been shown by a number of workers that just prior to birth or just after birth in various species those enzymes associated with anaerobic glycolysis become less prominent, while those associated with aerobic glycolysis become more evident. Anaerobic glycolysis becomes increasingly important during the last trimester of pregnancy and then starts to decrease very rapidly right after birth. As aerobic glycolysis systems start to become more significant just before birth, oxygen consumption of the cerebral cortex increases.

b. Enzymes associated with glutamic acid and glutamine synthesis begin to increase rapidly after birth. Thus, glutamine synthetase and transferase have been observed to increase dramatically in the kitten. Further, the levels of gamma-aminobutyric acid (GABA) in the brain also increase after birth, as do GABA transaminase (degrades GABA) and glutamic acid decarboxylase (converts glutamic acid to GABA). Associated with these changes is an increase of the free amino acid component of the brain, which is made up mostly (over 50%) by glutamine, glutamate, aspartate and GABA.

4. Chemical constituents.

a. Undefined lipids, neutral fats, cerebrosides, phosphatides and total sterols increase in man through the first 15 to 20 years, remain relatively stable until the age of about 50 years and then decrease in total amount.

b. Electrolytes. K increases with maturation while Na and Cl decrease, perhaps reflecting the decrease in extracellular water.

c. Protein increases in total amount during the first ten years in man and then decreases very slowly throughout the remainder of life. Total protein at birth is from 3.77 to 3.98% of fresh tissue weight. It increases to 8.99% at 35 years and then decreases to about 7.54% at 67 years of age.

(i) Amino acid incorporation into protein is very rapid during the growth phase of the neuron. Then, as the neuron reaches a relatively stable size, the rate of incorporation decreases rapidly and levels off as the growth rate levels off. Incorporation of labelled amino acids into protein occurs slightly more rapidly in the neonatal male rat, possibly reflecting the anabolic properties of testosterone.

(ii) During the first 105 days of life in the rabbit, it has been observed that the percentage of the protein present as globulin remains relatively constant while the amount present as albumin increases. This is reflected by an increase in the albumin:globulin ratio during development. Such changes may be associated with the suggestion that the half-lives of proteins synthesized in young animals are longer than those synthesized in old animals.

d. RNA changes with maturation have also been noted such that there have been observed to be changes in the quality of the RNA synthesized. This has then led to a change in the $\frac{G + C}{A + U}$ ratio, which was observed to increase with age in rats.

(i) There is also an increase in the total amount of RNA present with age as well as an increase in the RNA per g. This probably reflects in part the increase in Nissl substance in neurons with maturation. This finally decreases in old age.

e. DNA also increases per g with maturation and then finally decreases with advancing age. This would appear to reflect the increase in glial population during the early maturational phases associated with myelinization and finally the overall decrease in nerve cell number with advancing age. (The decrease in nerve cells with old age is not observed in all animals, for example, mice.)

B. Age changes. Age changes that are intrinsically those of the CNS are somewhat difficult to determine. There are clearly changes which occur in the brain with advancing age (neurofibrillar, amyloid body formation, argyrophilia, development of lipofuscin granules in neurons, etc.), but it has been difficult to ascertain whether these truly represent age changes which occur in the brain cells or whether they may be induced by age changes in the vascular system supplying the brain or be due to more generalized age changes in the vascular system which impair cardiac, hepatic, renal and gastrointestinal function and which then lead to changes in the nervous system. Binucleate ganglion cells have also been reported.

1. Morphologic changes (in man).

a. Gross atrophy is demonstrated by sulcal widening, decrease in brain weight, decrease in brain white matter and in nerve cell population density. The latter is clearly evident in the cerebellar cortex. Cortical neurons become smaller and lose their basophilic Nissl substance. In the cerebral cortex the greatest loss of neurons appears to be in the third cortical layer.

b. Accumulation of amyloid bodies in the regions just adjacent to ventricular or pial surfaces. These may be so numerous as to suggest that they may have some compressive effect on the surrounding nerve fibers.

c. Presence of senile plaques. These appear about the 6th or 7th decade and are usually found in the hippocampus and frontal lobe but may be anywhere in the cortex and in certain of the basal ganglia. They require silver impregnation to be visualized. They consist of argyrophilic material of a granular to filamentous nature scattered in a halo formation around an indefinite center containing a sudanophilic lipid or amyloid. They may be as small as 5μm or as large as 100μm in diameter. By electron microscopy they have been shown to consist of degenerating dendrites around a core of amyloid (Terry and Wisnjewski, 1970).

d. Neurofibrillary degeneration is found in the neurons of older people and consists of twisted coils of small tubules within the neurons. Many of these cells are surrounded by an argyrophilic-rich neuropil, which suggests that the primary change may come from the surrounding tissue.

e. Granulovacuolar degeneration is limited primarily to the hippocampus. The pyramidal cells become somewhat distended with vacuoles.

f. Astrocytes become more fibrous with aging, resembling in a sense the increase of fibrillar material which occurs in multiple sclerosis. Some of the protoplasmic astrocytes appear to accumulate a yellow, rather granular pigment. Glial fibers increase in the subpial zone, spreading more deeply into the cortex, particularly along the perforating vessels. There is also an increase in glial fibers in the striatum and globus pallidus.

g. Oligodendroglial cells show little change with advancing age, though there is an increased number of satellite cells around pyramidal neurons.

h. Lewy bodies are hyalin-like structures of uncertain etiology which are found in cells of the substantia nigra, locus ceruleus, facial, vagal and oculomotor nuclei. According to Greenfield, they may not be associated with aging in a senile sense, but are frequently observed in neurons undergoing degeneration.

i. Lipofuscin granules are pigment granules containing a pterin, which accumulate in many types of neurons in man, as well as in other species. They seem to occur more markedly in males than in females and to increase in accumulation in experimental animals on a vitamin E deficient diet. To what degree they interfere with neuronal function is debatable. However, as these granules fill the soma of a neuron and the RNA content of the cell decreases, one may wonder if they may not disturb some of the normal synthetic maintenance mechanisms of the neuron. Recent studies show these granules to be derived from lysosomes.

j. The leptomeninges are generally observed to become thickened with age, though this is not an invariable change.

k. The choroid plexus frequently becomes cystic.

l. Ventricular cavities enlarge as the number of nerves in the brain and their myelinated axons decrease in number, particularly in very elderly persons (hydrocephalus ex vacuo).

m. The pineal gland becomes filled with numerous calcareous granules with increasing age. It should be noted, however, that some of these are present at birth and there is no indication that this "brain sand" is in any way harmful.

n. The vasculature of the brain frequently becomes increasingly sclerotic with advancing age. Vessels are often completely occluded by this process, leading to areas of encephalomalacia. The internal elastic membrane becomes reduplicated or split into numerous smaller membranes and the media of the vessel wall undergo hyalinization. Collagen fibers continue to increase in number even after 60 years of age. The decreasing diameter of these vessels would appear to be of major significance in leading to aging of the brain (Kety and Sokoloff). It was noted that very elderly people without evidence of cardiovascular disease showed little or no sign of mental deterioration, whereas patients with such disease of the vascular system showed numerous indications of decreased mental acuity. Further, the arteriovenous oxygen difference was less marked in those persons possessing disease of the cerebral vasculature, indicating a reduced uptake of oxygen in such brains.

2. There are numerous biochemical changes with age which parallel some of those seen morphologically.

a. Reduced uptake of oxygen (associated with arteriosclerosis).

b. Glucose clearance from the blood also decreases with age. This occurs in persons whether or not they have cardiovascular disease.

c. There is a general reduction of all lipids, which parallels the loss of nerve fibers in the white matter. An analysis of the chemical composition of brain lipids indicates that their composition varies markedly with the age of the individual, being slightly different during almost every decade.

d. Both RNA and DNA increase in amount during the maturational aspects of aging and then decrease in total amount in old age (over 60 years). Further, the RNA base ratios change continuously throughout the maturational aging process. This suggests that the utilizability of the DNA code may be altered due to some effects on the repressor and derepressor substances of the nucleus. Such changes also are compatible with observations that the type of brain protein synthesized changes in older experimental animals, which were observed to synthesize more proteins of short half-life and fewer proteins of long half-life than younger animals.

Chapter 22

CASE HISTORIES

A. The following represent abbreviated case histories from patients seen in the hospital clinic or are histories constructed from observing the placement of lesions in autopsied brains. The student should first attempt to localize the anatomical components involved and the site (or sites) of the pathology and only secondarily attempt to identify the particular disease. A discussion of the cases follows at the end of the section on histories.

Case 1. Mrs B, a 39-year-old housewife, came to her doctor complaining of progressive weakness, first in her right hand and later in her left hand, of three months duration. On further questioning it was revealed that, before she had noticed any weakness, she had injured her right hand on two separate occasions. First, she burned her hand rather badly while ironing her husband's shirts, and two weeks later she cut her hand while peeling potatoes. On both occasions she felt no pain, and became aware of her injuries only on seeing her blistered palm and bloody hand.

On inspection, the metacarpal bones of both hands stood out clearly, suggesting atrophy of the intrinsic muscles of the hand.

Neurological examination disclosed loss of pain and temperature sensation over the thorax, and bilateral analgesia over the medial side of the hand extending to the midpalm, including the 5th and 4th fingers and medial aspect of the forearms and arms to the axilla. Other modalities of sensation were intact. Motor power was normal except for weakness and atrophy of the small muscles of both hands, with difficulty in abducting and adducting the fingers, adducting the thumb, or opposing the 5th digit. The cranial nerves were intact, and there were no gross reflex disturbances.

Case 2. A 60-year-old man was admitted to the medical service with the chief complaint of weakness and difficulty in walking. His past history revealed that he had had a complete gastrectomy (stomach removal) for a gastric ulcer five years previously. About two years prior to admission, he developed pins and needles, pains and numbness of his fingers and toes. About one and a half years prior to admission he developed unsteadiness of gait, stiffness of his legs and weakness in walking, with difficulty in walking becoming progressively more severe. He also complained that he felt tired and fatigued. His family claimed that he had become increasingly irritable lately, and had taken to checking the locks in the house frequently.

On neurological examination, he was a somewhat irritable man with a lemon-yellow tint to his skin. He had a broad-based spastic-ataxic gait. Romberg's sign was positive. There was a spastic paraparesis, with weakness especially pronounced in hip flexion, and in dorsiflexion of both feet. Deep tendon reflexes were hyperactive and equal in upper and lower extremities, with the exception of the ankle reflexes, which could barely be elicited. Abdominal and cremasteric reflexes were absent bilaterally, and there were bilateral Babinskis. There was impaired perception of light touch, pinprick and temperature over his hands and feet. There was loss of position sensation in both great toes, and of vibratory sensation at and below both knees. A laboratory analysis revealed severe anemia.

Case 3. Mr J, a 45-year-old travelling salesman had been suffering from sharp pains in both lower extremities for the past year, with pain becoming so frequent and severe in the past three months that he had had to consult a physician for relief. Before that, he merely felt a tingling sensation in both legs. For the past month he had been having difficulty walking, especially in the dark, and when walking in the light he had to watch the ground to keep from falling. Although he had had no actual weakness in his legs he tended to stagger and sway from side to side in walking.

On neurological examination his gait was observed as unsteady and broad-based, and he had to look at his legs in walking in order to keep from falling. A positive Romberg sign was present (inability to stand with feet together and eyes closed). Although there was no weakness or atrophy of the muscles, there was diminished muscle tone in all extremities. Deep tendon reflexes were markedly diminished in the upper extremities, and absent in the lower extremities. There were no pathological reflexes. Except for loss of position sensation in both great toes and absence of vibratory sensation below both iliac crests, sensation was otherwise intact. There was insensitivity of the Achilles tendon and testicles (Abadie's sign), and insensitivity of the ulnar nerve (Biernacki's sign). Pupils were irregularly constricted and failed to respond to light (Argyll Robertson pupil).

Case 4. A 40-year-old man was admitted to the hospital because of weakness and wasting of the muscles of both hands, difficulty in walking, with weakness of both lower extremities, emotional instability and slurring of speech.

Symptoms first began about a year prior to admission, with weakness of his right hand. Three or four months later, shrinkage of the muscles of this hand became apparent. At this time similar symptoms were noted in the left hand. About six months prior to admission he developed difficulty in walking, with weakness and wasting of the musculature of the lower extremities, more noticeable on the right. Shortly before admission he had been forced to remain in bed as he could no longer get about. In recent months the family had become aware of his exaggeration and prolongation of emotional responses, and of periods of involuntary laughing or crying. They also thought that his

204

speech was becoming less distinct and more slurred than normal.

On neurological examination, there was weakness and flaccidity of both upper extremities, especially distally in both hands, and weakness and spasticity of both lower extremities. Atrophy and fasciculations of the musculature of both upper extremities, and of the right lower extremity were present. Deep tendon reflexes were hyperactive and equal in the upper and lower extremities, with absent abdominal and cremasteric reflexes, bilateral ankle clonus and Babinskis. The jaw jerk, palatal and pharyngeal reflexes were hyperactive. The tongue was slightly smaller than normal, but was not wrinkled and had no fasciculations. Sensation was intact for all modalities. Marked emotional lability was noted, with a tendency to cry and laugh without sufficient provocation.

Case 5. A 14-year-old girl was hospitalized for the third time because of difficulty in walking. Five years prior to admission the patient noted an unsteadiness of gait, which worsened over the years until she was eventually confined to a wheelchair. She also complained of weakness and unsteadiness of her lower extremities. About three years prior to admission she developed some difficulty in manipulating her hands. Her parents also noted that her speech had become somewhat indistinct. There was a questionable history of neurological disease in the family.

On neurological examination she was found to have pes cavus (high arches) and scoliosis (curvature of the spine). She was unable to stand except with support due to unsteadiness, the unsteadiness increasing with closure of the eyes. There was weakness and flaccidity of both lower extremities. (On a previous admission there had been spasticity.) Deep tendon reflexes were moderately active and equal in the upper extremities, and markedly diminished in the lower extremities. Abdominal reflexes were absent, and there were bilateral Babinski signs. There was mild finger-to-nose ataxia and dysdiadochokinesis, with marked heel-to-knee ataxia bilaterally. Sensation was intact for all modalities except for impairment of position sensation in both great toes, and absence of vibratory sensation at and below both knees. Speech was slurred and syllabic or scanning in quality. There was horizontal nystagmus on right and left lateral gaze, as well as vertical nystagmus.

Case 6. A young man, aged 20, was referred to a neurologist with the following history. At the age of 18 years he had suffered an attack of subacute bacterial endocarditis, which had been treated with heavy doses of penicillin over a period of six weeks. About eight months previous to the present visit he had suddenly fainted and had been unconscious for several hours. Although consciousness returned, his mind was hazy for five or six days and he was not able to speak. Examination revealed spasticity in the right upper extremity, with loss of voluntary movement but no atrophy. There was no disturbance in the right lower or in either of the left extremities. On protrusion the tongue

deviated to the right, but there was no atrophy. The facial muscles below the
eye on the right were paralyzed. There were no visual defects nor somesthetic
disturbances.

Case 7. Mr J was admitted to the hospital following a fall outside his home.
He was notably undernourished, and seemed uncertain as to why he was in
the hospital. He claimed to be employed as chief of detectives for the FBI,
and described at great length the special case to which he was currently
assigned. This included a long recitation of a banquet the preceding evening,
which was given in his honor for recovering jewels stolen from a visiting duke.
When asked if he consumed much alcohol he admitted to an occasional drink.

On neurological examination, he was observed to walk with a wide-based
gait, and was unable to perform the finger-to-nose test or to run his heel
down his shin bone (bilaterally). There was impairment of position sensation
in the fingers of both hands and toes of both feet. There was impairment of
pain and temperature distally in both hands and feet in a glove and stocking
distribution. The strength of his wrist and ankle musculature was weaker than
that of the hip and shoulder joints.

Case 8. A 35-year-old man-about-town became slowly aware of some
disturbance in hearing in his right ear. Otolaryngeal examination demonstrated
that he had lost some hearing of all wavelengths of sound in the right ear, and
that he had nystagmus on lateral gaze. He commented that some months ago
he had been bothered by a continuous buzzing or ringing in that ear. Caloric
testing of the right ear produced no response, but induced nystagmus when
applied to the left ear. When asked to smile, it was noted that his smile was
somewhat pulled over to the left. He was unable to wrinkle his forehead on
the right side. Taste (sweet, sour and salt) was diminished on the right. The
corneal reflex on the right was diminished. Motor power and muscle tone
were normal elsewhere. There were no reflex changes in the extremities. There
was, however, right finger-to-nose ataxia. X-rays revealed a slight erosion of
the petrous portion of the temporal bone near the internal auditory meatus.
The precise site of his tumor is at the . . . .

Case 9. Mr C is a 55-year-old bookkeeper who was forced to give up his
position because of his inability to keep numbers straight. He complained of
left-sided headaches which were not relieved by aspirin. After many visits to
his local family doctor he was finally taken to see a neurologist when it was
observed by his family that his ability to understand verbal communication
was slowly decreasing, and that he kept repeating himself (perseveration)
when asked a question.

On examination, Mr C was observed to be well-nourished, but unresponsive
to questioning. His reflexes were within normal range, his cranial nerves were
all intact, and there were no sensory or motor deficits. Angiography revealed

a medial shift of the left middle cerebral artery, which was paralleled by a shift of his lateral ventricles to the right, as visualized by pneumoencephalography. A neurosurgical procedure was performed and a meningioma the size of a pullet's egg was removed. Within a month of surgery, Mr C's ability to communicate had notably improved. Identify the most likely site of the tumor.

Case 10. Case J injured his back, resulting in a fracture of a thoracic vertebra. Examination after treatment revealed loss of pain and temperature over the left side of the body below T_2, a spastic plegia of the right lower extremity and increased deep tendon reflexes in the right lower extremity, absent right abdominal and cremasteric reflexes and a positive right Babinski. The pupil of the right eye was constricted, there was enophthalmos on the right, pseudoptosis, vasodilatation and dryness of the skin (anhidrosis) of the right side of the face.

Case 11. Patient K is an elderly man with a history of diabetes of long duration. In recent months he developed frequent headaches and dizziness. One evening, following dinner, he became quite dizzy and momentarily lost consciousness. Examination after he had regained consciousness revealed left finger-to-nose and left heel-to-knee ataxia, loss of pain and temperature over the left side of the face and right side of the body, some difficulty in swallowing, with an absent gag reflex on the left, drooping of the soft palate on the left, with pulling of the left side of the soft palate to the right on phonation, hoarseness, nystagmus, with the fast component to the right and a left Horner's syndrome (miosis, enophthalmos, pseudoptosis, anhidrosis and vasodilatation). The sudden onset of symptoms suggested a vascular etiology.

Case 12. Mrs L, a housewife in her middle thirties, appeared in the doctor's office complaining of blurring of vision. Neurological examination revealed that her left eyeball was deviated outward and downward, that her left pupil was dilated and fixed to light and accommodation, and that there was a ptosis of the left upper lid. All other cranial nerves were intact. There was a spastic right hemiparesis, with increased reflexes and a positive right Babinski. There were no sensory changes, and no evidence of cerebellar dysfunction. The anatomical systems involved are the . . . . and her lesion would seem to be located in the region of the . . . .

Case 13. A similar case might be described in which all the symptoms would be the same except for those pertaining to the eye, which would be deviated inward, with normal pupils and absence of ptosis. The lesion in this case would be most likely to be at . . . .

Case 14. A third related type of case would again have the same symptoms for the extremities and trunk, but there would be no extraocular palsies or pupillary abnormalities. Instead, when the patient is asked to protrude his tongue, it would be observed to deviate to the left side and to be somewhat atrophic on the left. Fasciculations might be present. In this instance, the lesion would be at the level of the . . . .

Case 15. This patient, a man in his late fifties, developed neurological signs following a period of transient unconsciousness. On examination he was a moderately obese male with an arteriosclerotic appearance. Blood pressure was elevated. Examination of the visual fields by gross confrontation revealed a left homonymous hemianopsia. There was a spastic left hemiparesis, with deep tendon reflexes markedly increased in the left extremities, with absent left abdominal and cremasteric reflexes, a positive left Babinski and loss of pain and temperature sensation over the left side of the face and body, and of position and vibratory sensation over the left side of the body. The most logical site for this lesion is in the . . . .

Case 16. Mrs P also developed neurological signs rather suddenly over a period of a few minutes. For the past few years she had suffered from hypertension and arteriosclerosis.

On neurological examination, she was quadriplegic, with marked impairment of position and vibratory sensation in all extremities and trunk. Other modalities of sensation were unaffected. Cranial nerves were intact except for some questionable weakness of the trapezius and sternocleidomastoid muscles, which were somewhat flaccid. Her lesion would most logically be in the
. . . .

Case 17. In a third instance of neurological signs occurring after a sudden onset of unconsciousness, the patient was observed to have a bilateral hearing deficit in association with loss of position and vibratory sensation over the left side of the body. In this instance the lesion would most likely be located in the . . . .

Case 18. A patient with a bronchogenic carcinoma developed neurologic signs toward the end of his illness. Neurological examination disclosed a spastic right hemiplegia, with increased reflexes in the right upper and lower extremities, absent right abdominal and cremasteric reflexes, a positive right Babinski, a pronounced intention tremor of the left upper and lower extremities, and a left internal strabismus. A reasonable anatomical locus for the pathology would be in the . . . .

Case 19. A young woman was admitted to the clinic with a history of transient blindness in her left eye. This came on rather suddenly and cleared slowly over a two-month period. About six months later she suddenly developed a tremor of her left upper and lower extremities, a symptom which also appeared to regress with time. During her current admission, pertinent findings on neurological examination consisted of spasticity of the right lower extremity, with loss of position sensation and diminution of pain and temperature over the right side of the face. Can her problems be ascribed to a single lesion? Where would her lesion(s) be? . . . .

Case 20. A young boy of about 12 years of age was admitted to the clinic with a low grade fever, irritability, drowsiness, diarrhea, abdominal distress and headache. A few days later his temperature rose to 104 degrees (F) and he underwent a general collapse. When his temperature dropped he was noted to have paralysis of both lower extremities. Just preceding this phase his muscles were quite tender to palpation and flaccid. In the weeks following the paralysis, the muscles of both lower extremities became atrophic. There were no objective sensory changes, sphincteric difficulties or other neurological findings. The site of the lesion is the . . . .

Case 21. An elderly lady, whose relationship with her family had become somewhat strained due to her lack of involvement with the family and failure to help out around the house, was admitted to the hospital. Neurological examination revealed a masked facies, a weak, low and monotonous voice, and a face shiny and wet with perspiration. All movements were made with great effort, and she had great difficulty in getting up out of a chair. Posture was stooped, with flexion of the trunk, forearms and hands, and loss of associated movements of the upper extremities in walking. There was a rhythmical tremor (2—6 per sec) of all extremities at rest, with disappearance of the tremor during voluntary movement. There was marked rigidity and cog-wheeling of all extremities. The site of her lesion would be . . . .

Case 22. A patient was seen in the clinic with a type of abnormal movement which could be described as jerky and purposeless, but which frequently appeared to have a writhing character. The patient, who was 34 years old, had developed this syndrome during the past few months. His father, uncle, grandfather and several aunts all had developed similar symptoms by the fourth decade of life. The site of pathology would be . . . .

B. Review of case histories.

Case 1. The symmetrical loss of pain and temperature sensations on the medial aspect of the hands and the thorax suggests a lesion involving the decussating fibers transmitting these sensations from the side of entry to the opposite side of the cord where they would ascend in the anterolateral fasciculus. This would be in the region of the anterior white commissure of the spinal cord extending from about T_2 to T_1 or C_8. Since there has also been involvement of the intrinsic muscles of the hand, the lesion would appear to have spread into the ventral horn region at the level of motor supply to these muscles (syringomyelia).

Case 2. In this case the significant point is the gastrectomy without any apparent recourse to vitamin B_{12} therapy to prevent pernicious anemia. This has lead to subacute combined degeneration of the spinal cord with progressive degeneration of the posterior and lateral funiculi.

Case 3. Mr J is suffering from a disease entity which seems to produce its effect at the dorsal root ganglion cells first and then to influence the CNS somewhat later. The anatomical system involved is the fiber tracts passing through the dorsal columns. The sensations passing through the anterolateral fasciculus will also be lost due to the damage to the dorsal root ganglion cells. Finally, there is an interference with the sympathetic components which influence pupillary dilation resulting in an Argyll Robertson pupil (neural syphilis).

Case 4. This gentleman has a rapidly progressive degenerative disease which affects both the fibers in the descending corticospinal and corticobulbar systems and the motor neurons which provide for the final common pathway efferent impulses to the muscles. Though fasciculations were not noted in this patient, they are often present due to the slow destructive process of the anterior horn motor neurons. However, fasciculations are not noted as being present if the destructive process of the motor neurons is rapid, as in polio-myelitis. The disease process in this case is amyotrophic lateral sclerosis.

Case 5. This young girl is also suffering from a degenerative disease, which in her case has attacked the fiber tracts ascending in the dorsal column and in the spinocerebellar tracts. The cells of the nucleus thoracicus (Clarke's column) undergo degeneration. The pyramidal tracts appear relatively intact at the level of the brain stem, but become progressively involved as they descend in the cord. In some cases there may be loss of Purkinje cells in the cerebellum, as well as atrophy of the dentate nucleus and superior cerebellar peduncle. The middle peduncle has also been reported to show some involvement. Atrophy of nuclei and tracts in the lower brain stem has also been reported, involving the trigeminal, vestibular, glossopharyngeal, vagus and hypoglossal nerves. The disease entity is Friedreich's ataxia, a spinal form of hereditary ataxia.

Case 6. This young man is suffering from a thrombosis of a branch of the left middle cerebral artery in the region of the central sulcus producing the right-sided paralysis. (Patients with endocarditis frequently are left with diseased heart tissue from which a small portion may be broken away and come to lodge in some vessel as a thrombus.) It would appear that only a small area of cortex is involved, producing paralysis in the opposite hand and lower two-thirds of the face. The initial speech defect may be largely due to the edema surrounding the lesion and may or may not clear up, depending on how big the infarcted area is. More extensive loss of function on the right side did not occur as a result of the collateral blood supply from the anterior cerebral artery which has served to prevent a loss of blood supply on the lateral surface of the cortex to that part of the motor cortex innervating the arm and trunk.

Case 7. Mr J, with his history of hallucination and alcohol consumption, appears as an alcoholic patient suffering from a peripheral neuritis. This would appear to be the long-term effect of vitamin B complex deficiency, poor nutrition and the toxic effect of alcohol. Characteristically, his problems are both motor and sensory and are more marked distally than proximally. (It would be unlikely that such a peripheral distribution of symptoms would occur if he had CNS lesions. Further, the absence of pathologic reflexes (Babinski toe sign) in relation to his motor weakness also suggests peripheral disease.)

Case 8. The localization of a right hearing deficit, nystagmus, right facial paralysis, loss of sweet, salt and sour taste on the right and the reduced corneal reflex on the right and right-sided ataxia all suggest the presence of a mass in the right pontine angle (acoustic neurinoma). (An effect on the corneal reflex is common due to pressure on the trigeminal descending sensory nuclei.)

Case 9. The medial shift of the left middle cerebral artery and the lateral ventricle imply a space-occupying mass in the left hemisphere. The difficulty in handling numbers and inability to understand verbal communication also suggest a left hemispheric lesion, probably in the inferior parietal lobule, producing a receptive aphasia. This was verified at surgery.

Case 10. The symptoms listed in Case J suggest quite strongly that there has been a hemisection of the spinal cord at the T_1 level producing ipsilateral symptoms related to the dorsal column and lateral corticospinal tract and a loss of projection of pain and temperature through the anterolateral fasciculus which carries sensations entering the cord on the opposite (left) side of the body. Such a section of the cord also destroys descending sympathetic components terminating on the preganglionics of the first four thoracic segments. These give rise to ascending sympathetic trunk components which terminate in the face which when lost permit vasodilation, pupillary constriction and a loss of sweating. The eyeball also sinks into the socket as a result of a paralysis of the Müller fibers which normally suspend it.

Case 11. This patient has suffered an occlusion of the left posterior inferior cerebellar artery, producing the cerebellar ataxia in the extremities. This vessel supplies the dorsolateral quadrant of the medulla as well. As a result, the descending ipsilateral tract of the trigeminal nerve (pain and temperature) and the anterolateral fasciculus fibers (contralateral body pain and temperature) are lost. The tractus solitarius and its nucleus are also lost to produce the loss of the gag reflex, the difficulty in swallowing and drooping of the palate (nucleus ambiguus). The hoarseness is also related to loss of function of the nucleus ambiguus. The nystagmus may be due to a dyssynergia of the extraocular muscles or to a loss of function of the vestibular nuclei (Wallenberg's syndrome). Again, fibers of the sympathetic system pass through the area of involvement. The loss of these fibers produces the Horner's syndrome.

Case 12. Mrs L represents a case of an upper alternating hemiplegia in which there has been damage to the left oculomotor nerve at its exit to produce ipsilateral medial rectus palsy with external strabismus. There is also a compression or damage to those fibers in the pes pedunculi which form the lateral corticospinal tract passing to the opposite side to produce the right-sided hemiparesis.

Case 13. In this instance the patient is suffering from a middle alternating hemiplegia in which the level of injury is at the exit of the left abducens nerve. The destruction of this nerve, which supplies the lateral rectus muscle, leads to an internal strabismus. Again, the lesion compresses the descending corticospinal tract prior to its decussation to produce effects of an upper motor neuron disease contralateral to the side of the lesion; that is, that the paresis will be on the right side.

Case 14. This case represents the third variation of an alternating hemiplegia with the lesion at the exit of the left hypoglossal nerve. Inasmuch as there will be denervation of the intrinsic tongue muscles, there will be an observed atrophy on the side involved and the tongue will deviate to that side. As before, the paralyzed extremities will be on the opposite side.

Case 15. This patient, who has a number of neurologic deficiencies on the left side which developed over a short period of time, represents a patient with disease of the right middle cerebral artery affecting the fiber tract systems passing through the posterior limb of the right internal capsule (stroke with a capsular syndrome).

Case 16. Mrs P also presents as a patient with vascular disease. In this instance the vessel involved would appear to be a branch at the caudal end of the basilar artery or the rostral end of the anterior spinal artery supplying the region of the decussation of the corticospinal tracts and of the decussating fibers going to form the medial lemniscus from the nuclei of cuneatus and gracilis. A lesion at this site could readily produce a quadriplegia and quadri-sensory deficit.

Case 17. This patient is also probably a person with basilar artery disease. In this case it would appear that a small vessel supplying the pontine tegmentum in the region of the right side of the trapezoid body has become thrombosed. This would interrupt the decussating fibers from both right and left cochlear nuclei and the fibers of the right medial lemniscus as they pass through the trapezoid body.

Case 18. It seems most likely that this patient has developed a metastasis of his carcinoma with a small lesion developing in the basis pontis on the left side. This would interrupt the as yet undecussated corticospinal fibers to provide for the upper motor neuron symptoms on the right side. Since there is an internal strabismus, the level of the lesion would appear to be at the site of exit of the abducens nerve fibers. The intention tremor on the left side is related to the destruction of the pontocerebellar fibers. While it is true that the lesion would destroy pontocerebellar fibers going to both cerebellar hemispheres, which might be conceived as producing bilateral cerebellar signs, the symptoms are apparent only on the left because the tremors on the right side would be largely masked by the paralysis of the extremities related to the upper motor neuron disease on that side.

Case 19. The intermittent nature of this patient's symptoms, the combina-tion of early visual symptoms with long tract sensory, cerebellar and motor disease suggest that there are several lesions in the white matter, at least involving the cord and visual system (multiple sclerosis).

Case 20. The history of the events occurring in this patient resulting in a flaccid paralysis and atrophy suggest poliomyelitis with degeneration of the motor neurons of the ventral horn in the spinal cord.

Case 21. The characteristic masked facies, monotonous voice, wet face, stooped posture, difficulty in movement (rigidity) and tremor at rest all point to disease involving the substantia nigra (Parkinsonism).

Case 22. This patient is also suffering from what might be called disease of the basal ganglia, with there being primarily a loss of cells in the caudate nucleus and putamen. There are also areas of neuronal loss in the frontal cerebral cortex. Many of the remaining cells may be shrunken and filled with lipochrome. The abnormal jerky movements seem characteristic of those of chorea, while the writhing suggests some athetosis. The apparent hereditary nature of the patient's problems imply Huntington's chorea.

SUBJECT INDEX

218

Upper motor neuron 177, 178

Vagal fovea 36
Vagus nerve 10, 34, 166
Valium 180
Vascular system 85—108
Vasodilation 193
Vasomotor disturbances 193
Vasopressin 43
Veins 92—99
Venous sinuses 71
Ventral funiculus 175
Ventral horn 30
Ventral spinocerebellar tract 133
Ventricular system 109—114
Ventroanterior nucleus of thalamus 42, 173
Ventrolateral nuclei of thalamus 42, 170, 173
Ventrolateral reticular nucleus 34, 44
Ventroposterolateral nucleus of thalamus 42, 121
Ventroposteromedial nucleus of thalamus 42

Vermis 11, 40, 170
Vertebral artery 101
Vertebral-basilar arterial complex 85
Vertigo 167
Vesicles 4, 52
Vestibular connections 163
Vestibular nuclei 163, 165, 167
Vestibular system 40
Vestibular trigone 36, 37
Vestibulocochlear nerve 10, 34, 163
Visceral sensations 139
Visual agnosia 189
Visual pathways 145
Vitreous body 145—147

Wallenberg's syndrome 212
Wallerian degeneration 60
Water 196
White matter 45, 83, 199
White rami 191

Zona incerta 18